TIPS FOR FINDING HERBS USED BY CURANI
## CHAPTER 4: CURING THE BODY ............
UNDERSTANDING ILLNESSES ACCORDING T
THE CATEGORIES OF AILMENTS .................................................................. 42
ILLNESS MANIFESTATIONS ........................................................................ 43
HERBAL PREPARATIONS ........................................................................... 48
## CHAPTER 5: LIMPIA, OR SPIRITUAL CLEANSING .................................... 51
WHAT IS LIMPIA? .................................................................................... 51
HOW DO YOU KNOW YOU MAY NEED LIMPIA? ........................................... 53
HERB CLEANSINGS .................................................................................. 54
CRUCIFIX ................................................................................................ 55
CITRUS ................................................................................................... 56
FUMIGATION .......................................................................................... 57
EGG CLEANSING ..................................................................................... 57
## CHAPTER 6: CURANDERISMO AND EGGS .............................................. 59
EGGS AND HEALING ................................................................................ 60
HOW TO DO AN EGG CLEANSING ............................................................. 62
HOW TO READ AN EGG AFTER CLEANSING ................................................ 65
## CHAPTER 7: MAL DE OJO HEALING ....................................................... 68
WHAT IS MAL DE OJO? ............................................................................ 68
HOW TO PROTECT AGAINST MAL DE OJO ................................................. 70
WHO ARE MOST VULNERABLE TO MAL DE OJO? ....................................... 74
CURANDERISMO TREATMENTS FOR MAL DE OJO ...................................... 75
## CHAPTER 8: SUSTO HEALING – RETRIEVING LOST SOULS ................... 77
WHAT IS SUSTO? .................................................................................... 78
SUSTO AND CULTURE .............................................................................. 78
CAUSES OF SUSTO .................................................................................. 79
COMMON SYMPTOMS OF SUSTO .............................................................. 80
HOW MIGHT SUSTO BE CONFUSED WITH OTHER MENTAL ILLNESSES? ........ 81
PERFORM CURANDERO RITUALS .............................................................. 82
## CHAPTER 9: DAY-TO-DAY CURANDERISMO .......................................... 86
INGREDIENTS TO KEEP HANDY ................................................................. 87
ALTARS .................................................................................................. 97
TENDING TO YOUR ALTAR ....................................................................... 99

End of Year Routine ................................................................................ 99
The Day of the Messenger .................................................................... 100
How to Celebrate ................................................................................... 100
**CHAPTER 10: OTHER CURANDERISMO RITUALS ................ 102**
Curanderismo for Illness ...................................................................... 104
Kinds of Illnesses .................................................................................. 105
Forms of Treatment .............................................................................. 107
Curanderismo for General Wellbeing ................................................ 109
Spiritual Baths ....................................................................................... 109
**CONCLUSION ............................................................................... 111**
**HERE'S ANOTHER BOOK BY MARI SILVA THAT YOU MIGHT LIKE ................................................................................................. 113**
**YOUR FREE GIFT (ONLY AVAILABLE FOR A LIMITED TIME) ............ 114**
**REFERENCES ................................................................................ 115**

# Introduction

Have you ever been curious to learn about the ancient methods of shamans or how they used them to heal people from various ailments? Are you interested to learn about the world of Curanderismo? If that's the case, then read on. In the following chapters, we will introduce you to the fascinating world of Curanderismo and discuss the different healing methods. We will talk about how this holistic healing system originated and how it has changed throughout the course of history.

People have relied upon their local healers for thousands of years to ease their pain and suffering from various illnesses. Many cultures have used holistic methods that entailed restoring a person's inner balance to help them live a better life. It is not just about healing a certain part of the body that hurts. These systems aim to eliminate any negative energy that may have been caused by natural or supernatural means.

Traditional healers used what they had at hand, which generally meant creating herbal mixtures and concoctions from herbal teas to special ointments rubbed all over the body to promote better circulation. Each region is famous for certain medicinal plants, and these plants were used to heal people's minds, bodies, and souls for many years. Other techniques are further discussed in the following chapters, including massage, touch therapy, soul cleansing, and prayer rituals, among others.

Even though modern medicine does not acknowledge this type of healing, research scientists have discovered that the ancient herbs used by holistic healers from various cultures have proven to be medically effective. Through this knowledge, modern science was able to discover the healing properties of different plants used in regular treatments.

Whether you are interested in becoming a curandero or curandera or want to find out more about the world of Curanderismo, you have come to the right place. This book will show you the ins and outs of this magical world using a simple outline of each aspect of the practice. You will learn more about the important types of herbs and plants commonly used in Curanderismo rituals and treatments. You will learn how healers approach patients depending on their condition and learn their different healing methods.

In this book, you will discover the different types of ailments that can affect the human body, mind, and soul. You will also learn about the other methods and approaches that healers use to heal these different ailments. Learn about the history and origin of Curanderismo and how it has continued to develop to this day.

There will be various tips and tricks that you can incorporate into your daily life as you learn what you can do to maintain peace of mind. We will mention the best ways to choose a proper curandera or curandero; first, you'll need to get acquainted with the basics of Curanderismo. We encourage you to use the resources in this book to guide you in your journey toward learning everything there is to know about the world of Curanderismo.

# Chapter 1: What Is Curanderismo?

People of various cultures have developed holistic healing methods for thousands of years. These methods were not just aimed at relieving pain by treating one area of the body. They depended upon diverse approaches using medicinal plants and certain rituals to heal the person – physically, mentally, and spiritually. For many years, people used to visit their local healers to get rid of evil spirits or cure their ailments. In Central and South America, many countries practiced a type of folk medicine called Curanderismo. In this chapter, we will discuss the meaning of this healing and its different types, as well as give you a few tips on how to choose a proper healer or curandera.

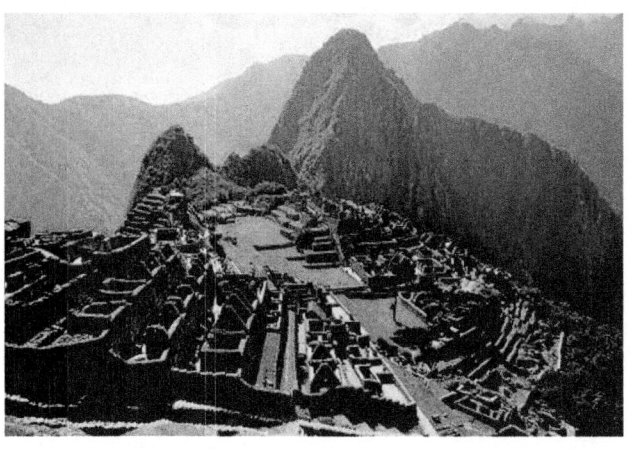

# The Definition of Curanderismo

Curanderismo is a type of folk medicine that has been practiced for hundreds of years in Latin American cultures. Since it is indigenous to Central and South American countries, the rituals and approaches used by the local healers are unique to that region. This practice mixes the use of herbal and medicinal plants with massage therapies and rituals that involve reciting a few prayers, which makes it a unique blend of beliefs. A healer will use a method that has been passed down through the generations from their ancestors.

The word is derived from the Spanish meaning of "cure" or "healing," translated from the word "*curar.*" The term "Curanderismo" refers to a method of holistic healing aimed at restoring inner balance and improving the quality of life. The healer who practices the ancient methods of Curanderismo is referred to as a Curandero (for a man) and Curandera (for a woman). However, the term may change depending on the region as it is practiced in several Hispanic countries such as Argentina, Honduras, Mexico, Guatemala, and Nicaragua. Some regions in the United States populated by people from Latin American cultures still practice Curanderismo to this day.

# The History of Curanderismo

The ancient cultures of the Mayans and Aztecs influenced this unique healing system. These cultures believed in a particular blend of religion and nature to sustain a healthy lifestyle. They thought that ailments manifest in the body when these factors are out of balance. This belief resembles Chinese holistic medicine, which involves resetting and restoring the flow of inner energy or Qi in a person's body. Holistic healing practitioners believe that to heal an illness, *you must be healed from the inside out.* This approach is different from modern or Western medicine, which usually only treats a specific organ or a symptom.

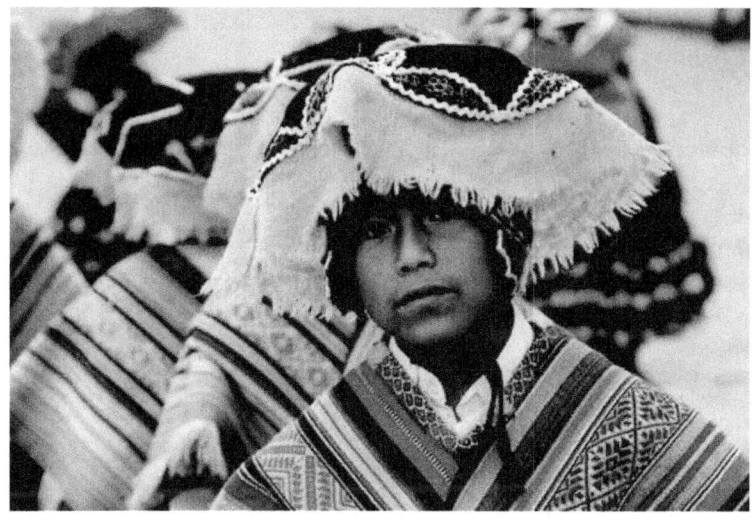

Holistic healers rely on botanical medicine that is to be found in nature. Knowledge of the healing effects of plants grown in each region has been passed from generation to generation. The Aztecs used to plant entire gardens with a wide range of medicinal plants that often numbered in the thousands of different species. Religious leaders would study the properties of each plant and document the experiments that were taught for generations.

Unfortunately, this documentation was destroyed when the Spanish occupation took place in the 1500s. Most of the gardens and research documents were damaged because science at that time was thought to contradict religious beliefs. However, people still remembered the characteristics of medicinal plants in these gardens, and the practice continues to be retold to this day. This knowledge has become one of the main pillars of the Curanderismo practice now.

At the beginning of the sixteenth century, the Spanish crusaders were fascinated by the ancient practices and healing powers of Curanderismo. One of the first Hispanic curanderos at that time was Alvar Nuñez Cabeza de Vaca. He was interested in the vast knowledge of the Aztecs and how they were able to cure people of various ailments using ancient knowledge of the medicinal plants of Curanderismo. He didn't have actual documents to learn from, so he started seeking experienced shamans to learn from them their traditional ways. The Indians considered Cabeza de Vaca to be a folk saint. They believed they would be immortal if they accompanied him in his healing journey. Many people wanted to become healers at that time.

Cabeza de Vaca combined his Catholic faith with the ancient Aztec knowledge of botany. His approach involved healing sick people by blessing them and reciting a few prayers over them, mentioning God's name. At the end of the treatment, they would make the sign of the Cross on the afflicted person. In the twentieth century, Cabeza de Vaca's teachings were passed on to Curanderos named Niño Fidencio, Don Pedrito, and Teresita. Many people approached these Curanderos as they believed them to be saints capable of magical powers of healing. However, their powers were not recognized by the Catholic Church.

The three Curanderos used different rituals for healing sick people. Fidencio specialized in medicinal herbal preparations in combination with medicinal baths people were instructed to be dipped in. He would then recite a few prayers while he conducted his treatment. Don Pedrito took the massage and touch therapy approach. Sometimes, he would use mud to rub on a specific body area that was painful to the patient. He also used herbal plants to brush the body from head to toe and provided holy water for people to drink to get rid of evil spirits. Teresita combined herbal concoctions with prayer and medicinal baths, but he innovated a bit by incorporating hypnotic techniques to heal people from their ailments.

The main teachings of Cabeza de Vaca strongly depended on his belief in God to cure all illnesses and drive away dark forces. He believed that religion played a major part in Curanderismo and that the patient's faith also influenced the healing process. Cabeza de Vaca used to heal Indians who did not share his Christian faith but believed in a higher power. His methods worked with them, which is why they idolized him.

The three Curanderos possessed charming qualities as they were excellent leaders, which is what attracted many people to them. They had hundreds of followers among common people and those in high places. Fidencio was able to heal the President of Mexico and his daughter, which, at the time, gave him high status and started a whole movement toward Curanderismo. Both Don Pedrito and Teresita had large followings among tribes. They all believed that their gift of healing came from God, which they felt was transferred to patients as they lay their hands on them. All of these Curanderos had common characteristics, and they were all considered folk saints because they healed sick people using herbs and special rituals while reciting prayers to receive healing powers from God.

Cabeza de Vaca was considered the first shaman of the movement of Curanderismo as he combined knowledge from the ancient world with the new world and Christian faith. After his time and that of the three Curanderos, many people learned the traditional methods of Curanderismo. After the departure of Cabeza de Vaca, a doctor of Aztec and Indian origin from Mexico City authored a book that included many medicinal plants but excluded a few that Cabeza de Vaca did not use but which were widely used by the Indians at that time. This book impressed the Spanish invaders who had thought the Aztecs were uneducated and incapable of possessing such vast knowledge.

Since the Spanish introduced the Christian faith to these lands, further influencing the practice of Curanderismo, this gave rise to a new form of healing, as healers began to recite prayers. At the same time, they conducted massage therapies or used therapeutic botanical preparations to treat sick people. Through time, many superstitions made their way into the practice of Curanderismo, as many cultures believed in witchcraft and evil dark forces that affect people's spirituality, which they believed could be manifested by mental or physical illnesses. The combination of all these rituals and medicinals shaped the healing system of Curanderismo to that which is practiced today.

# How a Curandero or Curandera Heals Ailments

People who practice and receive Curanderismo treatments believe that a body's illness may result from natural causes or supernatural evil forces. This is why many people prefer to visit a curandero or curandera to heal their spirits and drive these evil forces away, which cannot be fixed by Western medicine. A curandero uses herbal concoctions combined with massage techniques and prayer as they treat the afflicted person. People believe that many illnesses occur due to severe trauma that has led to emotional distress. A person may suffer from digestive issues, anxiety attacks, depression, loss of sleep and appetite, and an overall sensation of indifference. This prevents them from enjoying life, and these symptoms are believed to affect their spirit negatively.

A common symptom caused by emotional trauma is *bilis,* which is attributed to extreme anger and rage. A person usually suffers from headaches, indigestion, nausea, vomiting, weight loss, constant fatigue, and, in extreme cases, fainting, coma, and even death. The physical explanation, in this case, is that the person usually has a lot of trapped bile in their system. Another disease that affects the digestive tract is called *empacho*, which happens when an indigestible substance is trapped in the digestive tract, which leads to clogging.

A curandero or curandera would have the person lie on their stomach while they massage their back in a specific way. At the end of treatment, the healer would pinch the skin above the tailbone until they heard a snap, indicating that the substance blocking the digestive tract had passed. The patient may also be given a special herbal tea to help dislodge the indigestible material from its place and promote better circulation. Another malady comes about when it is cold, which affects the stomach and which leads to colic, which is then treated with mint tea.

Many different types of plants were used for thousands of years to heal ailments using Curanderismo methods. Recent scientific research has found out how these plants are medically effective. For example, aloe vera was used as a soothing agent to treat cuts and burns in ancient times. Today, aloe vera is known to treat bacterial infections and inflammation. Many of the plants used in ancient medicine have been found to have curative effects in today's world.

Curanderismo is also used to help ease the suffering of people who undergo chemotherapy. A treatment session by a curandero or curandera is given to alleviate the adverse effects of this particular cancer treatment. It is also used to cure mental ailments such as chronic anxiety, depression, and post-traumatic stress disorder. Curanderismo is also performed to relieve emotional trauma and distress in women who have had stillbirths or miscarriages.

Other types of sickness are believed to be a direct result of witchcraft practices, which usually manifest in mental diseases more than physical ailments. Witchcraft and sorcery target a person's spirit and are thought to cause most of the more dangerous ailments. These are usually the toughest to recover from and require an experienced curandero or curandera to drive away the evil spells and dark forces from a person's spirit. The effects of these illnesses manifest in a person's psyche as they may experience frequent nervous breakdowns, emotional distress, melancholy, chronic anxiety, paranoia, depression, and even schizophrenia and other dissociative disorders. The patient may also experience hallucinations or delusions leading to suicidal behavior.

To practice Curanderismo, the healer must believe strongly in their ability and healing powers. These powers are believed to be gifted to certain people from God. Curanderos or curanderas usually pray in the names of the spirits of saints to help them connect with their inner healing ability. This is so that they can channel these powers to heal ailments or drive evil forces away. A curandero or curandera may use different treatment methods depending on the severity of each case. Their treatments may include spiritual cleansing or limpia to heal afflicted spirits. They may also use a few tools and props such as candles, essential oils, double-crosses, holy water, herbs, eggs, spices, and certain flowers and fruit. Each item is used for a specific treatment according to the type of ailment.

Curanderos or curanderas usually use Holy water and candles to absorb evil energy and protect the patient against them. There are different types of candles for each purpose. For example, a red candle is lit in a room to promote strength, and a blue candle is lit to provide harmony between family members and other people gathering in a room. Some herbs are tied in a bundle and brushed on a patient's body from head to toe to avert evil forces and negative energy. A common technique entails using a raw egg that is rubbed against the body to absorb the negative energy of the evil eye or *mal de ojo*. Other plants like garlic are also used to divert evil spirits.

Another common practice is using a sweat lodge, which many people in the Western world use today, and which is now known as a *sauna*. A curandero or curandera prepares a closed heat hut or a *temazcal* by creating a steam flow by pouring water over hot stones. This practice is used for various treatments, from promoting relaxation and cleansing the skin by opening up the pores to respiratory healing issues and cleansing people's spirits. Many healers also use humor to make people laugh during their therapy sessions, which helps release endorphins responsible for making human beings happy and help release tension and stress.

There are other treatments available to people experiencing emotional distress. A curandero or curandera may instruct a person to dig a hole in the ground and then proceed to let out all of the repressed feelings and negativity they have been experiencing in their lives. People sometimes become hysterical during this treatment as they scream out their emotions. As they continue with the process, they gradually calm down as they release all that trapped energy. The healer then asks the person to cover the hole to bury their troubles and negative feelings. Many people swear by this method and believe that is where the term "bury your feelings" originated.

## What Are the Types of Curanderos or Curanderas?

There are three main types of healers who practice the ancient methods of Curanderismo. The first type is a healer who mainly uses herbal plants with medicinal properties in most of their treatments. This type of healer is called *Yerbero,* and should be an expert in choosing the right herbs, plants, flowers, or fruit to treat specific illnesses. A Yerbero uses herbal tea or topical concoctions. Some are in the form of medicinal ointments, pastes, or creams to be applied on certain areas of the skin. Some of these herbal preparations are burnt to drive away evil forces or avert negative energy.

The second type of healer is called a *Partera,* who is usually the local midwife and is knowledgeable in types of magic related to birth. Pregnant women visit their Partera to drive away any negative energy that may affect the baby's health (or the mother's) or to ensure a smooth birth. Other women may visit a Partera to help them get pregnant if they have suffered from regular miscarriages. On the other hand, women who don't wish to get pregnant can also get help from a Partera to avoid accidental conception. A Partera also uses methods to help new mothers heal faster after delivery. She also has various treatments for women's reproductive organs.

The third type of curanderos or curanderas specializes in massage techniques where they touch specific points in the body to cure various diseases. This technique is also popular in Asian culture, especially in Chinese culture, which uses acupressure and acupuncture techniques on specific pressure points in the body to restore inner balance. All three types of healers follow the same concept in Curanderismo, using herbs, rituals, prayers, and touch techniques to heal the body, mind, and soul from various ailments.

## Modern-Day Curanderismo

Curanderismo is still a popular practice today among Hispanic groups in North America and many countries in Central and South America. Many people still believe in the healing powers of this holistic system as they believe it is a kind of complementary treatment they need to seek in combination with modern medicine. For many years, Curanderismo was the only medical practice available to various cultures, and many of the older generation believe in its power to this day.

While older generations strived to keep the ancient tradition of practicing Curanderismo alive, people today fear that the practice may disappear because today's younger generations don't believe as strongly in traditional practices faced with the alternative of modern medicine. However, Curanderismo is still widely practiced. The most common teaching method is a direct transfer from parents to their children in each generation. Suppose a person wishes to learn everything about Curanderismo. In that case, they need to be trained by an experienced curandero or curandera, who has regularly practiced Curanderismo over a long period of time.

Curanderismo practitioners usually conduct their treatments in their own homes. This approach creates a private place that encourages better communication between the curanderos or curanderas and their patients, which, in turn, creates trust as the core of their Curanderismo techniques. The healer needs to get in touch with the patient's suffering to understand what they are dealing with. Many believers would like doctors today to integrate modern scientific and medical knowledge with ancient holistic healing methods such as those used by Curanderismo. However, modern-day medical professionals don't acknowledge this holistic healing system. It is thought that the teachings of Curanderismo will begin to disappear in the upcoming years.

## How to Choose a Proper Curandero or Curandera

The process of choosing a proper practitioner of Curanderismo is crucial. You need to do extensive research about the world of Curanderismo to get an idea of what to look for. There are many online courses available that teach and certify Curanderismo practitioners. Some workshops can take as little as two weeks to get you certified as a healer. However, this is not what you should be looking for. You have to be aware of a few aspects before you decide.

The best and easiest way is to find personal referrals like from a friend or family member who has tried treatment at the hands of a curandero or curandera. If you can't find any referrals, you should research online for local healers in your area. Based on people's reviews, narrow down your search to two or three healers maximum. The next step is to interview each one of them. Many healers may have a busy schedule and can't meet with you at short notice, so it is best to contact them via email or text or through their website if they have one.

In your email or message, mention why you are seeking treatment from a curandero or Ccurandero by writing a little about your pain.

Then, ask them a few questions. The most important thing in a professional healer is experience and knowledge. Your first question should be, "How long have you been practicing Curanderismo, and where have you obtained your knowledge?" It is important to note that it takes many years for a person to become a curandero or curandera. Make a comparison column to list all the attributes of each healer so that you can decide which way to proceed.

The next question is about the approach they plan to take with your treatment. As discussed previously in this chapter, there are three types of curanderos or curanderas. Depending on your type of ailment, you'll need a specific kind of treatment. Ask your potential healer why they think that approach is the best way. It is good to get concurrence from the other healers as well.

Sometimes, you may find two or three healers with almost similar experience and knowledge. If that is the case, then you need to follow your intuition. You must be comfortable with your healer and not just choose them based on experience and knowledge. When you enter a treatment room, and you're willing to completely surrender to the healing powers of a healer, you are more likely to have a good experience and become healed. Be as picky as you want when choosing your healer. Give the matter a lot of thought, just like anything important to you.

In this chapter, we introduced you to the world of Curanderismo and its history through to today. We discussed the various methods that curanderos and curanderas use in their treatments and the three main types of healers. The upcoming chapters will explore in greater depth more aspects of this holistic healing system to give you a wider view of what happens in this fascinating world.

# Chapter 2: The Three Realms – Mind, Body, and Spirit

As is the case with nearly all forms of alternative medicine worldwide, Curanderismo is a complete health solution for the people who follow it. Like traditional Chinese medicine and many forms of African medicine, Curanderismo is based on the premise that the body is only happy and healthy when all components are properly aligned and there is harmony between the body, mind, and spirit. The problems that people face, whether they are mental problems, physical or spiritual problems, Curanderismo aims to heal through holistic treatment and a well-rounded approach.

While Curanderismo is generally seen as a Mexican or Mexican-American form of healing, some other philosophies are integrated into the discipline. Originating from Spanish-speaking regions, there is a heavy influence from Mayan, Aztec, and Spanish Catholic religious ideas. How a curandera or curandero approaches a problem depends largely on the kind of beliefs they hold and the kind of curandera training they receive. As you move around in the Southern American countries such as Mexico, Guatemala, Peru, and other regions, you will notice that the way Curanderismo is carried out will start to change. Depending on the popular local religions and what kind of history they have experienced, different practitioners will manage problems in their own unique ways. Even though there can be differences in the diagnosis and treatments between different practitioners, the underlying philosophy is usually the same.

## Treatment Philosophy

In some regions, there is also an African influence in medicine and remedies, and these teachings have significantly influenced the local population of that area. Naturally, these things flow into the work of the curandera. While curandera is used for nearly every medical problem, it is more popular as a treatment for spiritual and mental problems and those diseases that are not being cured by traditional medicine.

If someone has a cold or a fever, these are things that can easily be cured through standard western medicine practices. Moreover, these treatments are not very expensive. They are quite easy to find as conventional doctors will be able to help you with this kind of problem. However, when things get slightly more complicated, as is the case with problems such as diabetes or cancer, modern medical treatment tends to get far more expensive and also starts to become varied and sometimes vague. There comes a point where you are just trying different treatments, but nothing is really happening. In some cases, western medical interventions have either had a very bad effect or have not remedied the situation, causing people to move away from it altogether.

Many people claim to have found a cure for serious problems such as cancer and have even been able to change their destiny with the help of a seasoned Curandera.

Practitioners of Curanderismo are very well-respected individuals in their societies, and in many cases, they are even leaders. Generally, being a curandera is seen as a skill and blessing given only to certain people; not all of them can assist others with the same level of effectiveness. Many curanderas believe that healing is something inherent in the nature of humans and that everyone has some kind of healing skill within them. The main challenge is to tap into these skills and learn how to harness them to benefit others.

## Specializations within Curanderas

Like modern medical science, curanderas can also specialize in certain things. For instance, some people help to treat physical ailments, some practitioners specialize in metaphysical problems, and others deal with things like destiny and bad luck.

At the most basic level, there is the Yerbero, who is a person who specializes in herbal medicines. These can be prescribed for something as common as the seasonal flu to something as complex as cancer or hepatitis. Their strategy for treatment usually relies on some consumable medicines in the form of teas and basic pills or through ointments or creams. They may also have dietary recommendations to be followed and may also suggest some edible herbs and plants to help resolve the problem.

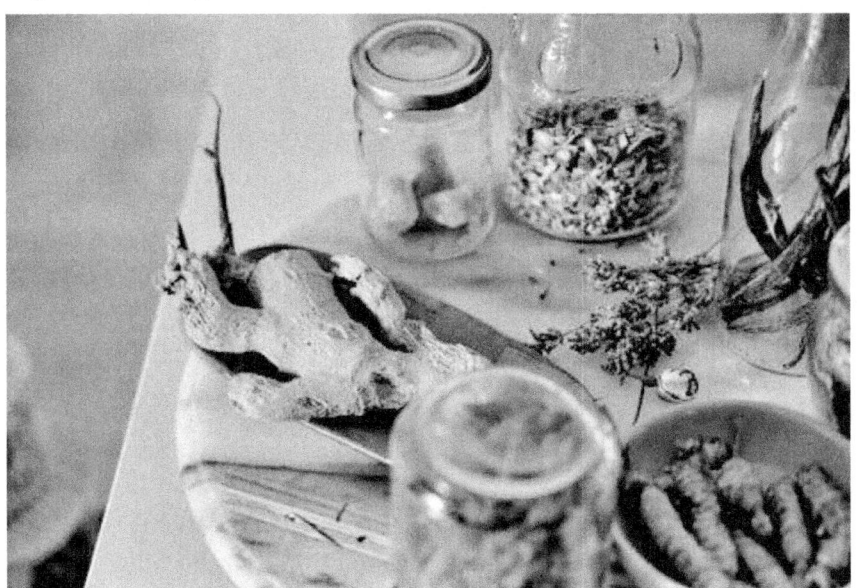

The Partera is a practitioner who specializes in matters related to childbirth – and also magic. This role can be described as being similar to a modern-day gynecologist. This healer can help a woman if she is having trouble with pregnancy, assist during the entire pregnancy period, help with childbirth, and also help with postpartum care. The Partera is the specialist to see for any problems related to the female reproductive organs.

The final stage of treatment is found with the *Espiritualista*, the medical expert for spiritual problems. These practitioners help people overcome all kinds of personal and metaphysical challenges. This could be something such as not being able to sleep properly and being a borderline insomniac, to things like hypertension, depression, and anxiety. These experts can also be consulted regularly (simply to talk to) and they will evaluate whether the patient is doing well mentally.

Overall, the specialists can be grouped into those that help with problems on the physical level, those who help with mental problems, and those who assist in spiritual issues. However, in all tiers of treatment, the practitioner will nearly always take a holistic approach and try to address all facets of the person to relieve them of their problem. Curanderos see health and illness as the result of the interaction between the mind, body, and soul. This could translate into being the interaction between a person's religion, their emotional condition, and their physical condition, resulting in a problem. However, this does vary depending on the client and the kind of treatment that the practitioner decides to offer. For instance, if a person is not religious at all but the practitioner follows Catholic Christianity, the situation will be very different compared to a patient who is also a religious person and a practitioner who uses the traditional religious beliefs of the Mayans.

However, in all situations, the curanderas make extensive use of symbolism, much like how it is often used in modern psychology. The tools and how the symbolism is used will vary from one situation to another and between one practitioner and another. For instance, some practitioners prefer to have the patient bathe in water and wash physically to achieve spiritual cleanliness or experience a rebirth. On the other hand, there is the temazcal ceremony in which practitioners make a small tent, a bit like an igloo, and fill that space up with steam by pouring scented water over hot volcanic rocks. Then the patient goes into this tent, spends a few moments there, and then crawls out of it (imitating what a person does when they are born), and eventually achieves a rebirth and starts afresh.

## Healing the Spirit

A lot of the problems that people solve through the assistance of a curandera are problems that have a metaphysical origin. Things like curses, mental challenges, problems in life, and many other issues are all seen as problems encountered due to destiny, through the natural course of life, or as a result of magic and spells. The spells and magic are known as Brujos and are something that have no solution in western medicine. For some problems caused by spells and magic, the curandera has to perform a *barrida* ritual. This is a process in which the affected person is treated to cleanse them of negative energy and help them get a fresh start. The way practitioners perform this cleansing does vary, though, and, in most cases, eggs are used to absorb the power of the negative energy, and then these contaminated eggs are moved away from the affected person.

Two of the most common problems that people seek help for are the evil eye and a situation known as susto, which is characterized by problems such as depression, insomnia, stressfulness, and anxiety.

The evil eye is a situation that babies are very prone to. It is usually triggered when someone looks at something with envy, jealousy, hatred, anger, or any other extreme and negative emotion. The consequence is that the child, or the person, may have an accident, they may have a series of negative events that never seem to end, or they may experience financial loss or any problem as a result of negative situations. All of these things start to happen for no apparent reason. This is something that is also seen in many other cultures, and there is no medical explanation for it. However, holistic healers, spiritual healers, and various forms of traditional medicine do recognize this as a problem, and they have a treatment for it.

To cure a person of the evil eye, the curandera will use a mixture of physical and spiritual exercises. As mentioned above, some practitioners will use eggs to draw the negative energy out of the patient, while others will also add the use of the herb rosemary to brush the patient with and metaphorically cleanse them of the negative energy. Using a few branches of rosemary, they will brush their head, torso, and limbs and try to brush away the negativity that is causing all of their problems.

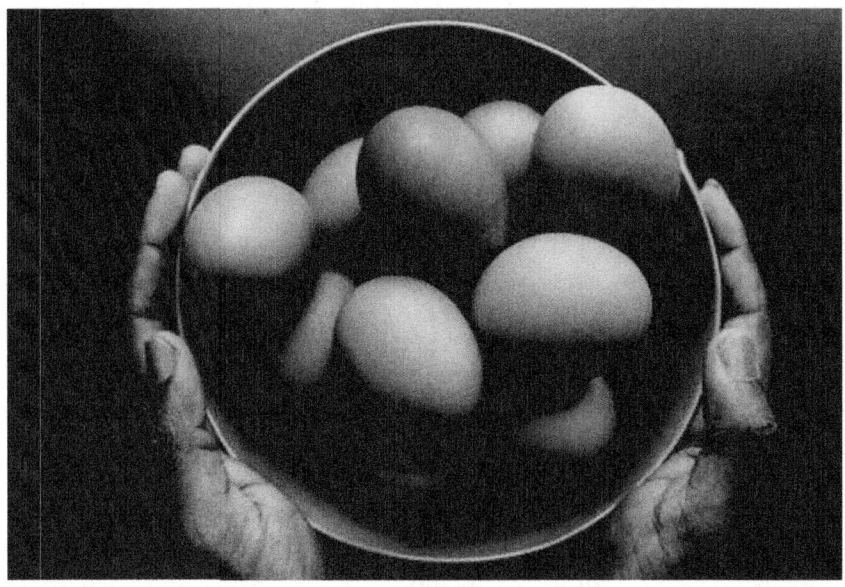

Similarly, the egg is also rubbed over the body, and this is meant to draw all the negative energy out of the body. After this process, some experts will break an egg into a glass of water and study the condition of the egg in the water. Based on its structure and the condition of the egg, they will even make predictions about the future of the patient and will also offer suggestions on how that person can protect themselves in the future. During the entire process, practitioners may chant prayers, there may be some religious singing, or the practitioner may recite some verses from a holy book. Again, because this form of treatment draws from so many different cultures and religions, there is no single book or single doctrine that is followed. Depending on the school of thought they follow, they may use books from any of the Abrahamic religions.

## Healing the Body

Curanderismo makes use of naturally occurring ingredients to formulate all kinds of treatments for physical ailments. These cover every imaginable physical problem. However, not all practitioners have the expertise to treat every kind of problem. In fact, some curanderas specialize in certain problems, such as skin issues, reproductive problems, and specific diseases such as diabetes or cancer. Herbs and plants are used extensively to help to cure patients. These can be used in the form of teas; they can be consumed as they are, or they can be used to make herbal medicines.

Curanderas also use a lot of aloe vera and give garlic and onions special importance as well. These items are used in different ways to cure people of diseases through the use of garlic, and onions are also used by other healers who are attempting to heal mental problems or spiritual problems. In some cases, the practitioner may suggest a person should either increase or decrease their intake of onions and garlic to facilitate the healing process. In this form of treatment, the practitioner may also suggest the use of certain fruits. One very popular treatment is papaya juice therapy which is used to help heal digestive problems. Today, through science, we are beginning to understand that the gut and brain connection is one that has a significant impact on the overall performance of the body. Through this traditional Mexican treatment, people have not only experienced a better gut, but they have also experienced changes in their mood, sleep, memory, and focus. Moreover, papaya therapy is also used to treat patients who suffer from mental problems, especially if they are suffering from sleeping problems or bad dreams, and this therapy has been shown to be very effective.

Similarly, the use of aloe vera has been part of therapy used for centuries in Curanderismo, specifically for skin problems and things like cuts and burns. Today, modern science also tells us that aloe vera has some amazing health benefits for the skin and hair. More importantly, some of these plant-based therapies are also used to counter metaphysical problems. For instance, if a person were having negative spiritual experiences or was facing any kind of intangible problems in their lives, they would be advised to place an aloe vera plant at the entrance of their home.

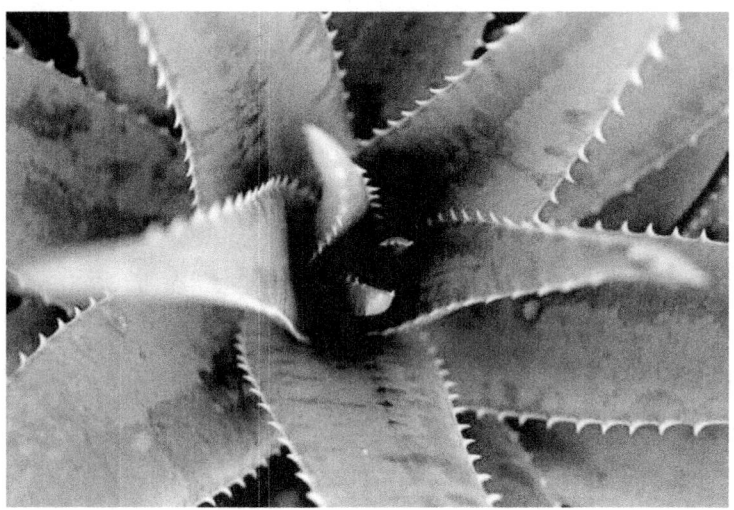

Vera plant

Animal-based medicines are also used a lot in this form of treatment. This can include things such as oil derived from various organs of different animals, snake oil that is derived from the skin of snakes, and various other liquids, creams, and powders that are created using different parts of certain animals. Moreover, animals and various plants and herbs are also used in different ceremonies that are performed to treat patients. As mentioned earlier, rosemary is used quite commonly to cleanse people, while there are other plants or herbs often burned during ceremonies to benefit from their smoke, energy, or aroma.

In some cases, the ceremonies have to be done in the presence of a Curandera, but in other cases, the guide can teach a patient certain movements and exercises they can do on their own. One of the very common therapies in Curanderismo is the shawl or towel therapy that is used to assist pregnant women. During the pregnancy, the mother goes through a lot of discomfort when the baby is in an odd posture, and this may strain her body. By tying shawls or towels around the hips of the mother and around her lower back, practitioners can maneuver the baby in the womb. In this way, they can help the baby get into a different posture and get out of a position that may be harmful to the mother or the child. Usually, the child is supposed to move around in the womb and is meant to turn on a frequent basis. If this isn't the case, then shawl therapy can be quite helpful in this process. This therapy also comes in handy if a woman is experiencing pain after the delivery. In some cases, the mother may feel pain for several months after the delivery or even years after delivery. However, due to intense changes that the body goes through, such as the opening of the hips and the change in the spinal structure, this can be a very serious problem to deal with. Even in these cases, shawl therapy can be used to help bring the body gently back into its correct position and reduce the pain.

Some of these therapies, such as the temazcal therapy discussed above, where the person goes into a hot rock tent and crawls back out to imitate rebirth, are regular therapies that a person can do on a frequent basis. Even if a person isn't suffering from any medical problems, doing this can be a great way to release stress from the body and make sure that they are filled with positive energy all the time. Many people regularly attend these therapy sessions and experience different benefits, from physical benefits such as an increased heart rate, open pores, and better breathing to more spiritual and mental benefits such as feeling more relaxed, feeling more positive, and not feeling so burdened by life's worries.

One of the most effective therapies found in other traditional treatments is laughter therapy. This is something that patients can do on their own or in a group with or without a leader. The concept is very simple, and everyone gets together and laughs out loud. Modern science now shows us that laughter releases endorphins, and this creates a wave of benefits for the body. Higher endorphins do everything from improving our immune system to helping our body fight off infections to helping us sleep better by increasing oxygen flow throughout the body. Moreover, the presence of endorphins in the body helps protect us from stressors and makes it possible for us to take things head-on rather than always being worried about the consequences.

Another very effective strategy that is used for both mental and physical wellbeing is the concept of burying your problems. During this therapy, a person will literally dig a hole in the ground and start to talk about all of their worries and apprehensions and problems over the hole and then fill it back up with soil. Whether it is a traumatic experience that you are unable to get over or you are just worrying about the future and find it hard to sleep at night, everything and anything can be said, and all you have to do is cover it up with soil. This is a great way for a person to release pent-up energy and negativity and externalize all of this emotion through a very physical process. This process has been shown to have a range of physical, mental, and spiritual benefits for the people who practice it.

In all of these processes, it is important that a patient has a good connection with their healer. Even if this is a situation where the healer isn't physically present, and the patient is just working from instructions the healer has provided, having a positive relationship with the healer is very beneficial.

# Chapter 3: Key Herbs and Plants

*DISCLAIMER: These medicinal plants should never replace conventional medicine. If you believe that you may have a medical issue, first and foremost – visit a specialist. Do not ingest any plant that might contain toxic elements.*

In this chapter, we will be discussing some of the most common herbs and plants used by curanderos. These are the herbs that have been shown to have a significant effect on humans in their rituals. We'll explain what they do spiritually and how they can be used by a curandero, as well as provide one or two tips on how to find them.

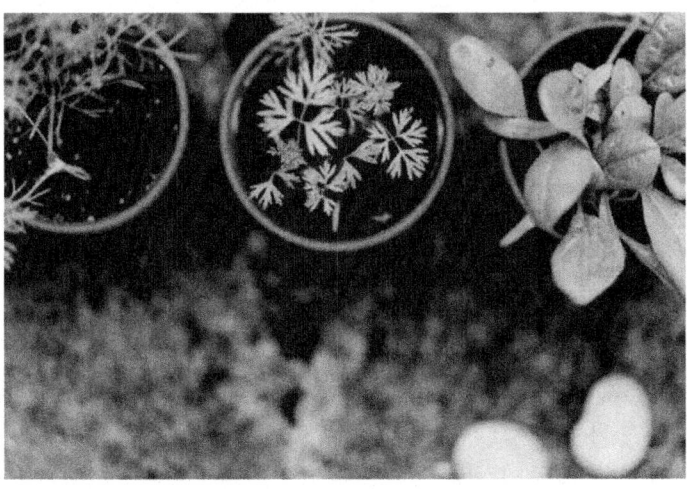

# Importance of Herbs and Plants in Curanderismo

Curanderismo is a healing system that integrates traditional Mexican and ancient Mesoamerican spiritual practices. Curanderos (healers) use plants, animal parts, minerals, and other methods to heal their patients. These treatments may include herbs such as aloe vera leaves for burns or for moisturizing the body after taking a steam bath. Dried marigold flowers are used to heal bruises and soothe aching muscles. Mexican oregano can be used to prevent infection of wounds, and drinking chamomile tea can be useful when you have trouble sleeping.

Most of these practices have been passed down for generations, making Curanderismo an integral part of Mexican culture.

Herbs and plants play a large role in Curanderismo as they are abundant, inexpensive, and widely available. Herbs can be found growing wild or cultivated on farms throughout Mexico. They are often used to make remedies, teas, and ointments for a wide range of illnesses. Some plants are eaten or crushed into juice form to treat certain conditions such as indigestion or stomach aches.

Herbs are important in Curanderismo because they provide inexpensive treatments that anyone can access regardless of their financial status. While Western medicine may be expensive, herbal remedies are available to anyone who is willing to search for them.

Curanderos use plants in their practices because they see the spirit of the plant as an integral part of its healing power. The belief that "like cures like" plays a role here; if someone has respiratory problems, using an herb or plant that is known to cause respiratory discomfort (through allergies or other negative effects) may provide relief.

If someone has a headache, drinking herbal tea made from plants known for their pain-relieving abilities can help reduce the severity of the headache. The spiritual beliefs behind this treatment lie in the idea that all vegetation contains spirits and can be used as a medium to communicate with the spiritual realm.

In some cases, plants may be used in a form of divination to let curanderos know what kind of treatment is needed or if they are even on the correct path toward healing their patient. Sometimes this can result in an herb being mixed into a remedy which helps heal one ailment but may cause another.

Some plants are believed to provide spiritual benefits. Chamomile, marigolds, and other flowers may be worn or carried by patients to enhance their mood or help lift depression. Herbs containing caffeine (such as maté) can act as stimulants helping patients stay awake if they suffer from fatigue.

Curanderos also use plants for their beauty treatments. Flowers are often added to baths, worn as garlands or wreaths, or burned to cleanse a space energetically and spiritually.

Herbs can be used through teas, poultices, lotions/oils/salves, creams and gels, and other topical applications for physical healing. They can also be used for spiritual healing by being burned or by releasing their fragrance into the air.

Herbal remedies often provide non-invasive options which do not cause side effects or interact dangerously with other medications. This is a major benefit of Curanderismo as it provides people with an alternative to Western medicine's sometimes-toxic treatments.

## Common Plants and Herbs Used in Curandero Spells and Rituals

There are many different common plants and herbs used in curandero spells and rituals. Although there isn't a set list of what must be present for the ritual to work, some believe that certain types of plants have specific magical powers. Here is a small list of common plants, with examples:

### Ambrosia Arborescens or Ragweed (Marco)

Marco is a plant native to the Andes Mountains and has been used for centuries. It is usually burned to cleanse a ritual space, but it can also be an added ingredient in spells or rituals involving purification, protection, love magic, and more. The leaves and stems of the plant have been used as an anti-inflammatory, pain-relieving, and antiseptic for centuries.

### Baccharis Salicifolia or Mule Fat (Chilca)

Baccharis salicifolia is a blooming shrub native to the sage scrub biome and desert southwest of the United States, northern Mexico, and parts of South America. Chilca has been used as a traditional medicine for treating inflammation, stomach pain, and insomnia due to its curative effects. This plant's medical qualities represent an important source of pharmaceutical chemicals.

### Brugmansia Sanguinea or Red Angel's Trumpet (Guanto Rojo)

The Red Angel's Trumpet is a species of tree that grows in the Andes Mountain Range between Colombia and Ecuador. It has been used as an entheogen by the South American Indians for thousands of years. Brugmansia sanguinea contains poisons in all of its parts. So, beware! Treating Angel's Trumpet as a drug, especially by smoking it or making some sort of concoction with the plant, is extremely dangerous and can be fatal.

### Citrus Medica or Citron (Limón)

The Citron is a lemon-like citrus fruit that has been around since ancient times. The plant can be used for any type of traditional medicine, and it was commonly found in Roman baths because the citron possesses antibacterial properties to heal wounds, making it an excellent natural antiseptic treatment.

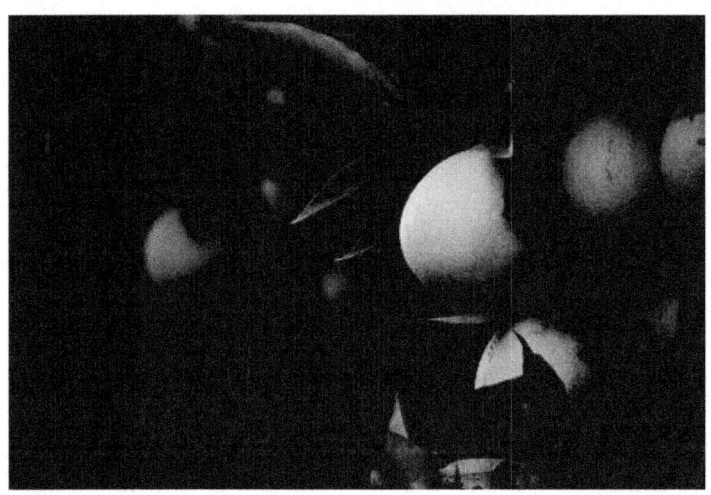

The citron has been valued for its medical purposes since ancient times. It is useful for combating respiratory problems, intestinal disorders, seasickness, scurvy, and other diseases. The antibacterial essential oil of the flavedo (the layer of rind) has also been used in traditional medicine.

Curanderos often use this plant as an ingredient in their healing spells by rubbing the rind all over the body.

**Dianthus Caryophyllus of the Carnation Flower (Clavel)**

The Carnation flower is a sweet-smelling, edible flower that has been around since the sixteenth century. This plant is one of the most commonly used by curanderos, and it can be found in many different types of spells such as love magic, protection from evil spirits or bad energies, and even for relief from anxiety.

They are edible and sweet-smelling flowers that have been used in traditional medicine for centuries. The spiritual meaning of Carnations symbolizes a celebration of love, abundance, and joy.

For Shamanic treatment, the patient is usually soaked in a bath full of carnations.

### Eucalyptus Globulus or Eucalyptus (Eucalipto)

This ultra-powerful antibacterial treatment is used to heal any type of wound or infection. The plant is also used to cure body aches, relieve pain, and heal burns or scars.

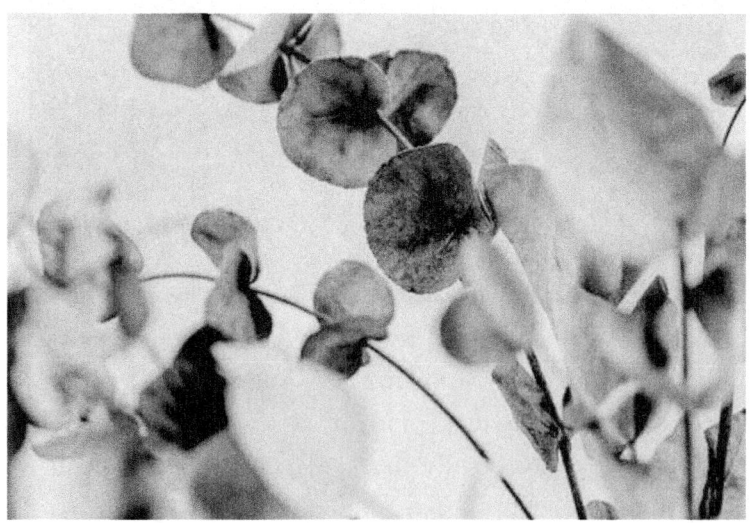

The medicine comes in the form of a steam bath additive made up of eucalyptus leaves boiled in water for about twenty minutes before applying it on your skin like an ointment that will leave you feeling refreshed in no time at all!

This plant is also used as a natural insecticide.

A patient's body is usually brushed with a branch of eucalyptus leaves and stems, or vaporized eucalyptus oil is used to heal the patient.

The leaves and stems of the plant have been used as an anti-inflammatory, pain-relieving, and antiseptic for centuries.

### Mentha Piperita L. or Peppermint (Hierba buena)

Peppermint, an aromatic herb, has been used for centuries to treat nausea, vomiting, indigestion, and stomach pain. The plant also helps with asthma attacks by providing relief from common colds or respiratory problems.

The oil is used in aromatherapy as a flavoring agent, and the leaves can be consumed via tea or infusion.

It is also great for repelling mosquitoes, so you might want to carry some peppermint oil with you if you decide to go camping during mosquito season!

Hierba buena essential oils are used by curanderos to repel evil spirits and negative energies.

### Mentha Spicata or Spearmint

Spearmint is a strong-scented, aromatic plant that has been used by many cultures for thousands of years. This herb can be found in spells to break bad luck or remove negative energies and black magic from your life.

The leaves are crushed into teas or infused with water, producing an oil full of vitamins and minerals that is great for the skin.

Curanderos use Spearmint to treat indigestion, nausea, or vomiting by boiling a few leaves in water before drinking it as tea.

### Minthostachys Mollis or Tipo

Minthostachys Mollis is a South American Andean medicinal shrub restricted to Peru, Colombia, Venezuela, and Bolivia. Curanderos rub a patient's body with the plant's leaves to remove evil spirits or bad energies.

The plant is prepared as a tea and used therapeutically as an aphrodisiac and carminative in Andean indigenous medicine practices.

### Nicotiana Tabacum or Tobacco (Tabaco)

Tobacco is a common ingredient in many curandero spells and rituals. The plant has been used for hundreds of years to remove negative energies or illnesses caused by black magic, hexes, curses, bad luck, or even evil spirits.

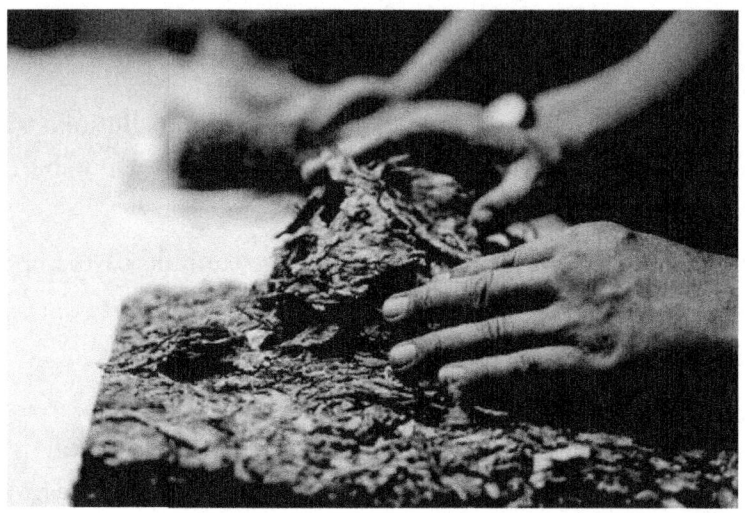

The leaves are usually crushed into ethereal extracts, which can be applied to the body to break hexes or curses.

Tobacco is harmful to the body and should not be ingested.

### Prunus Serotina or Black Cherry (Capulí)

The black cherry is a strong-scented plant that grows in many parts of the world. The fruit, bark, and leaves are all used to make medicine.

Curanderos use the black cherry plant to neutralize any sort of negative energy or hexes.

It can also be used as an expectorant for coughs and colds.

### Rosmarinus Officinalis or Rosemary (Romero)

Rosemary is a shrub with fragrant evergreen needle-like leaves and purple flowers.

The plant has been used for thousands of years as an essential oil, tea, or infusion. It can be added to your bath in order to remove negative energies from your body.

Other medical uses for rosemary include its anti-inflammatory properties, increasing memory and concentration, or assisting with muscle pain or stiffness.

### Ruta Graveolens or Common Rue (Ruda)

Rue is a plant with sharp-smelling leaves and yellow flowers. The herb has been used for thousands of years to remove negative energies or hexes from the body.

Curanderos use rue in their spells by crushing it into ethereal extracts, burning its branches on coals, or mixing it with water before applying it topically.

## Everyday Plants Used as Medicine in Curanderismo

### Garlic

Garlic is used both as a food and medicine (it is also called poor man's penicillin). Garlic contains phytochemicals, such as alliin and the enzyme alliinase. These chemicals give garlic its characteristic pungent taste and odor. Allicin has been found to be an antioxidant with anti-clotting properties that may protect against cardiovascular disease. Alliinase is a sulfoxide that can be converted to oxidized allicin, which has been found in studies on garlic and cancer prevention to have potential anti-cancer activity.

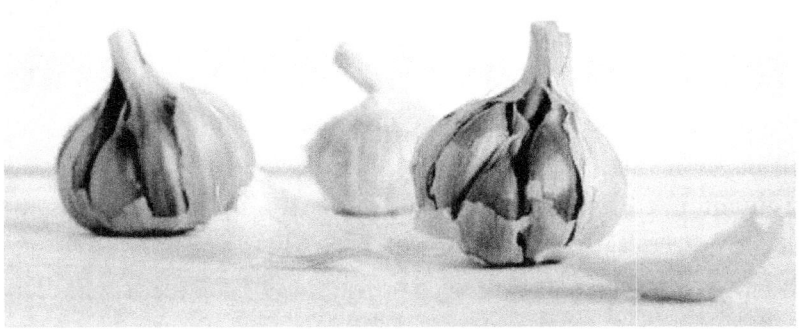

### Onion

Onions are a food source containing antioxidant properties. Onions may also have some preventative benefits against cardiovascular disease, cancer, and asthma. It is believed that the antioxidant and anti-inflammatory properties of foods such as onion may prevent cancer by inhibiting oxidative damage to DNA. Studies have also reported a reduced risk of several common cancers, including lung, stomach, and colon cancer.

### Cinnamon

Cinnamon is a spice used in cooking but has been found to potentially help reduce blood sugar levels when added to the diet. Cinnamon is also used in Ayurvedic medicine for stomach complaints, including indigestion and constipation.

### Ginger

The active constituents of ginger are its volatile oils (gingerols) which comprise about two percent of fresh weight. Ginger has been found to potentially benefit nausea associated with pregnancy, chemotherapy, motion sickness, and morning sickness. Ginger has also been found effective in preventing the symptoms of rheumatoid arthritis. The anti-inflammatory activity of ginger is related to several therapeutic properties, including inhibition of inflammatory enzymes such as cyclooxygenase (COX).

### Turmeric

Turmeric, one of the primary ingredients used in curry powder, is believed to be anti-inflammatory and antioxidant. There are some current studies on the potential health benefits of curcumin (the active constituent in turmeric), including its role as a dietary supplement for cancer prevention. It may also have beneficial effects against Alzheimer's disease by preventing amyloid-beta peptide accumulation.

### Green Tea

Tea is one of the most widely consumed beverages worldwide. Green tea, in particular, possesses high concentrations of catechins and possesses potent antioxidant properties that have been shown to be protective against cardiovascular disease. Researchers are studying potential anti-cancer benefits from green tea's polyphenolic compounds (flavonoids). The effects may also include an inhibitory effect on platelet aggregation and smooth muscle cell proliferation.

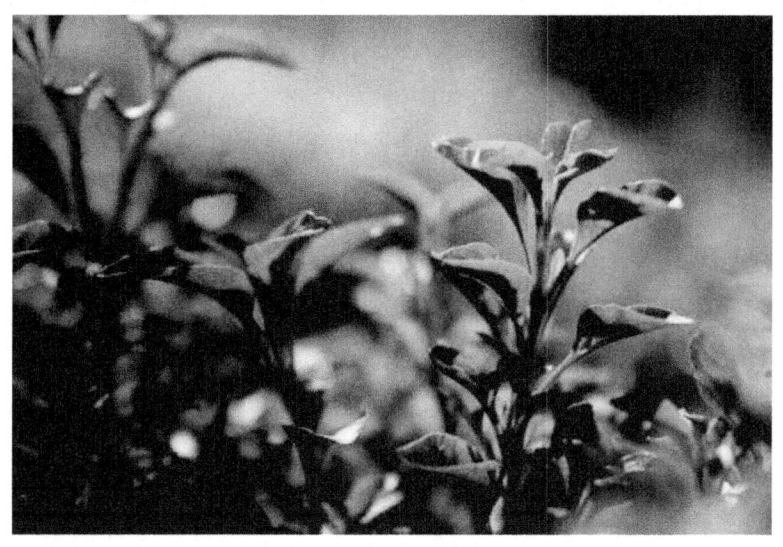

### Coffee

Studies have found that coffee consumption is associated with a lower risk of type II diabetes, Parkinson's disease, and liver cancer. Coffee also contains antioxidants (chlorogenic acid) which may provide cardiovascular benefits by inhibiting low-density lipoprotein oxidation and reducing blood pressure. Coffee also contains caffeine (a stimulant) and theophylline, which have been found to potentially provide anti-inflammatory benefits by inhibiting pro-inflammatory mediators such as lipopolysaccharides and COX enzymes.

### Cocoa

Studies indicate that cocoa may be a rich source of flavonoids with antioxidant activity that may protect against cardiovascular disease. The cocoa plant also produces the stimulant methylxanthine (caffeine).

### Chocolate

Chocolate is made from fermented and roasted seeds of cacao tree pods native to South America. Chocolate contains many potentially beneficial compounds, including catechins, polyphenols, caffeine, and other methylxanthines.

### Red Wine

Wine is derived from the fermentation of grape juice and contains many potentially beneficial compounds, including resveratrol, catechin, epicatechin gallate (ECG), quercetin, tyrosol, and hydroxycinnamic acids such as caffeic acid and ferulic acid. The grape seed extract is also a source of proanthocyanidins which have been reported to possess antioxidant and anti-inflammatory properties.

### Aloe Vera

Aloe vera is a cactus-like plant native to Africa and the Arabian Peninsula. Aloe has been used by many civilizations throughout history as both an ornamental garden plant and for its medicinal properties and nutritional value. The leaves can be cut or torn open so that the gel inside may be consumed raw or applied topically.

## Risks of Using Herbs and Plants without Knowing Their Properties

The risk of using an herb or plant without knowing its properties is that you may harm yourself. Most herbs and plants are dangerous if they aren't used properly, especially when performing spells or rituals, because you can easily mess up the dosage, for example, which could have negative consequences. One must first learn about how to identify the plant before using it. It is also important to learn how it can be used and what the right dosage is for its intended purpose.

Modern medicine does not allow the use of herbs and plants, as several reports of toxicity have been identified. Hence it is critical to know the properties of a certain plant before using it.

Ingesting an herb or plant without knowing its properties can be dangerous.

We recommend that you search for a practitioner of Curanderismo, if possible, to guide you through the process.

There are many plants and herbs which have been used in sorcery, witchcraft, black magic, and spiritual healing over thousands of years throughout history by indigenous people from different regions of the world. However, most of the time, it is not safe to use them without knowing their properties. It is always better to work with a Curandero who knows how these plants are used and what you should do for everything to go well.

## Herbs in Western Medicine vs. Curanderismo

Western medicine and Curanderismo have a completely different approach when it comes to using plants. In Western medicine, doctors know exactly what kind of plant they are prescribing because the dosage is very precisely measured for each medicine created. Traditional healers may not necessarily be as precise in their dosages, which can vary from person to person, and it is possible for one to take too much or too little, which could have negative consequences for the patient.

Curanderismo is a healing tradition that has been used by indigenous people across the world and throughout history, but nowadays, there are several reports of toxicity associated with some herbs because not everyone knows how to identify them correctly. If you are interested in learning how to use herbs for your own benefit, then it is always better to find a Curandero who uses traditional methods and who knows what they're doing.

In Western medicine, scientists have found that there are some plants that can be used as remedies, while others can cause more harm than good depending on the dosage. On the other hand,

Curanderismo has been used for thousands of years, and there are various plants that can be helpful in certain situations. However, one must learn how to identify them first before using them because it is possible for someone to take too much or not enough, which could have negative consequences like toxicity.

## Tips for Finding Herbs Used by Curanderos

There are some plants that can be found in most regions of the world, but others only grow in certain places. It is important to learn about where they grow so you know what an herb is supposed to look like before trying your luck at finding it because there could be several environmental differences between one place and another, even if it is the same species.

Knowing what season is best to harvest the plant is also vital because some plants only grow in certain seasons, so you should avoid harvesting them until it is the proper time, or you could kill them off without realizing it.

Curanderos usually use these herbs because of their powerful spiritual properties when used correctly during rituals and healing practices. It can be very dangerous for someone who doesn't know what they're doing to try and use them without supervision from a Curandero.

In this chapter, we've provided you with a list of some of the common plants and herbs used by curanderos for their spells and rituals. We also gave you one or two tips on how to find them in your area if they aren't growing near you already. As always, make sure that you are careful when harvesting any plant from nature, as there may be other creatures that depend on those plants for survival. Ensure that you know which plants to pick and how much you need. If in doubt, consult a curandero for their advice.

# Chapter 4: Curing the Body

*DISCLAIMER: These medicinal plants should never replace conventional medicine. If you believe that you may have a medical issue, first and foremost – visit a specialist. Do not ingest any plant that might contain toxic elements.*

Curanderismo is used to cure various illnesses of the body, mind, and soul. We've already discussed the most important medicinal plants and herbs used by Curanderos and Curanderas; in this chapter, we'll discuss how traditional healers use botanical concoctions in combination with other therapies to treat different ailments.

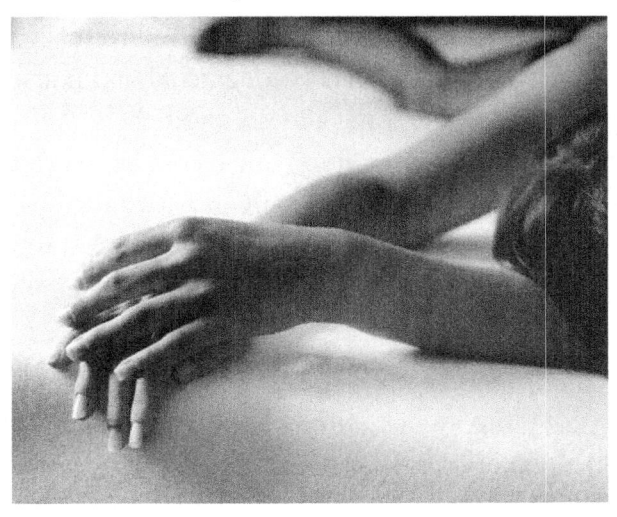

# Understanding Illnesses According to Curanderismo

A core concept of Curanderismo is that any type of illness is caused by an imbalance in the body as a whole. This imbalance happens more often than not when a person is affected by excess heat or cold in their body. The treatment approach taken by the curandera or curandero entails using herbal concoctions and other types of therapies -accompanied by a few prayers to help restore balance in the body.

Richard Currier thoroughly explained this idea in the 1960s. He explained that this imbalance is first introduced to people's bodies as children when they are weaned from their mothers. The child interprets the weaning process as a rejection from the mother, who has stopped providing the source of nourishment.

This rejection becomes associated with feelings of withdrawal and being cold, which are opposite to what the child was feeling when he/she was receiving regular nourishment from the mother. These feelings remain with us as we grow older. This is known as the hot-cold syndrome, which is responsible for how we contract illnesses and how we cure them.

In Curanderismo, the traditional healer would usually use various approaches to restore the balance between cold and hot sensations in the body. They associate some illnesses with heat and others with cold. An illness may be caused if too much cold air enters the body or if the body overheats. Illnesses that happen as a result of cold entering the body include headaches, earaches (commonly known as *aire del oido* or air in the ear), chest and stomach cramps, teething, paralysis, rheumatism, and tuberculosis.

A chest cramp occurs when the body has a fever and the person breathes in cold air. Aire del oido is exactly what it sounds like, which is when cold air enters the ear, causing an earache. A headache occurs when cold air enters the head, similar to how earache is caused. A stomach cramp usually occurs when the body is warm and the stomach catches a draft of air. This happens especially when you are wearing light clothes in cold weather. The process of teething is associated with cold illnesses because the teeth that are pushing through the gums are considered to be cold.

As for illnesses associated with heat, these include sore eyes – which you get when you have strained your eyes by focusing too hard while working. It is also believed that when your feet are cold, blood travels upward to your head and eyes, which also causes them to overheat and leads to eye strain. A sore throat is also believed to occur as a result of cold feet – in a similar way to sore eyes. Dysentery is also a hot disease as it leads to the release of blood in the stool. This disease may be caused by eating a lot of hot food. Kidney diseases are considered hot illnesses, and they are usually accompanied by symptoms of fever, swollen or red palms, and itchiness in the feet. Teeth infections and abscesses are a result of accumulated blood in the tooth's root, which is also considered a hot disease. Any other irritations or inflammations that occur in the body are considered hot diseases like having rashes, acne, and warts.

Some diseases can happen as a result of either hot or cold, like diarrhea. If it is associated with cold, it will produce a loose stool, and if it is hot, it will produce a green stool. Severe diarrhea may lead to an inflammation in the small intestine called enteritis and can also affect the stomach and large intestine. The hot type of enteritis is associated with bloody stools, and the cold type is associated with mucous discharge.

While toothache in the molars is considered a hot disease, pain in any other tooth is considered a cold disease.

A cold is caused when the body is susceptible to entry into the cold air, especially when it is warm. On the other hand, a hot ailment is produced from the body itself. When heat originates from the body, this is more dangerous than when the body is exposed to excessive heat from the outside. Your stomach is the most heated region in the body, which makes it most susceptible to a cold disease. When the feet are exposed to the cold for long periods of time, the heat travels to the throat and head. Hot and cold illnesses mainly affect the digestive tract. To achieve proper balance and maintain good physical health, a person should not eat too much food that is either hot or cold.

## The Categories of Ailments

In Curanderismo, the category of illnesses is diagnosed, and treatment therapy is instituted through careful study of the cause of the illness and not just the symptoms. There are two types of illnesses, which are natural and supernatural. The natural ailments (or *males naturales*) occur as a result of an imbalance of heat and cold in the body. The supernatural ailments (or *mal puesto*) occur when people are affected by dark forces from witchcraft and sorcery. The treatment of natural ailments involves restoring physical balance by removing excess heat or cold from the body. On the other hand, treating supernatural ailments requires the extraordinary powers of a curandero or curandero, which is used to remove or divert the dark forces away from the body. In supernatural ailments, a person may be exposed to spells by witches or negative energy from evil spirits. Mal de ojo or the evil eye is a cause of supernatural ailments.

The teachings of Curanderismo entail having a strong faith in God to protect you from evil spirits. Many people follow traditions that revolve around family and being an active member of the community. These traditions are practiced within the framework of religion, which is one of the pillars of Curanderismo. To maintain good health, a person needs to be in balance physically and spiritually.

# Illness Manifestations

## Caida de la Mollera

This type of illness affects the soft regions of the head. *Caida de la mollera*, or fallen fontanel, usually affects babies whose skulls are still developing. It takes around 18 months for the front fontanel to close. If a baby falls on its head, this will lead to a depression in the upper palate of the skull, which will block the oral passage. This may lead to other symptoms like diarrhea and fever, and the baby won't be able to breastfeed.

The treatment usually consists of treating the depressed region in the skull. A curandera or curandero will carry the baby facing upward while reciting certain prayers, such as the Ava Maria. The healer then proceeds to push the upper palate up with their thumb three times while reciting the prayers. Simultaneously, the healer pulls the baby's hair. An alternative is to fill the baby's mouth with water as the healer sucks the depressed palate on the skull to restore its shape.

In extreme cases, the healer will break an egg and take the egg white and yolk to rub it into the baby's hair. The process is repeated as many times as possible to retain the shape of the skull. At the end of treatment, the healer holds the baby upside down by the ankles and shakes the baby three times. Another way is to carry the baby sideways and then shake the body to allow blood flow to the head. The baby's feet are tapped three times in the end. The treatment has to be done swiftly by the hands of an experienced practitioner because this is a serious condition causing a blockage of the oral passage, which means that it does not allow food to be properly digested.

## Empacho

This is another type of illness that mainly affects children but has been found to occasionally affect adults as well. Empacho is characterized by a blockage in the intestinal tract, usually from an indigestible food like gum, *which children often swallow*. Regularly swallowing gum can lead to the formation of a large mass of gum that sticks to the intestinal or stomach wall. The apparent symptom is a swollen ball-shaped mass in the stomach. It is normally found in children under the age of two years, who will usually throw up as soon as they eat anything because it cannot be digested. Other symptoms include diarrhea, fever, and major discomfort. A healer diagnoses empacho by examining the child's calves for small knots or masses.

To treat empacho, a curandera or curandero employs massage and touch therapy in combination with the use of an ingestible herbal blend. The child's stomach and back are rubbed downward with oil to facilitate the movement of the food through the digestive tract. The healer simultaneously pinches the lower back sideways to lengthen the constricted muscles to create a straight pathway for the food to pass. The herb used in this treatment is *hoja sen*, which is dried and mixed with cotton. The mixture is then burned and added to milk, which is given to the baby. This mixture is designed to break down the hard mass of food so that it passes down through the intestinal tract. The child may experience discomfort in the abdomen, so the healer gives them another drink made by boiling milk with white sage. The child is then left to rest, and the body must be kept warm to recover.

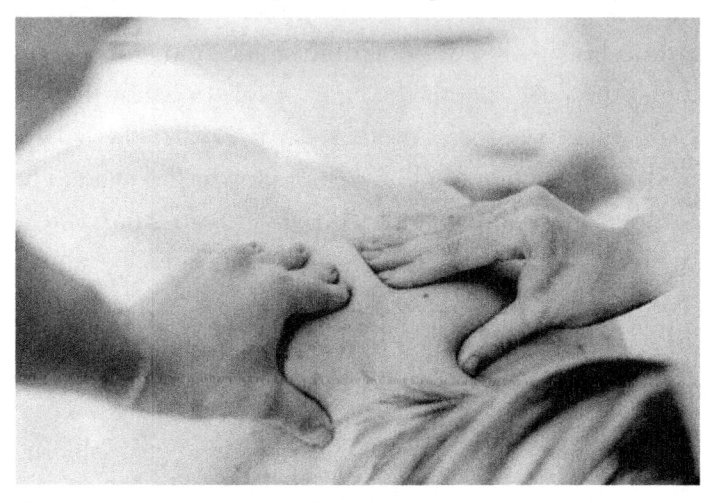

Another treatment for this ailment includes massaging the stomach and then rubbing it with a raw egg. The egg must be kept at room temperature. At one point, the egg bursts in a certain spot in the stomach, which indicates the location of the empacho. A piece of cloth is tied around this area, and then the child is given castor oil to drink to facilitate bowel movements.

Empacho is usually diagnosed by using a special pinching technique. The healer pinches the lower back and listens to see if there is a snap sound. This makes it easier to differentiate empacho from other digestive tract illnesses.

### Susto

Susto is another form of natural illness and refers to natural fright that may affect a person. It may bear a resemblance to another condition (called *espanto)* - a spiritual or emotional scare. Susto refers to the emotional distress that people feel after experiencing trauma. This may include signs of PTSD, stress, anxiety, depression, loss of appetite or sleep, and chronic fatigue. A person suffering from susto may lose all interest in doing anything even if it is something they previously enjoyed doing.

A curandero or curandera is able to diagnose a person with susto by taking their pulse, and if it is irregular, chances are they are suffering from susto. In advanced stages, the disease is called *susto pasado*, and the patient experiences excessive coughing and fatigue. They may even experience epileptic seizures as they have flashbacks to a previous traumatic experience. A person may have susto after an accident, miscarriage, and loss of a loved one, among other serious emotional experiences. They might suffer from susto if they were in a distressful situation. For example, if a person is claustrophobic and was trapped in a closed space for hours, this might be a consequence.

In Curanderismo, it is believed that when a person is suffering from susto, their soul leaves their body. The person's essence becomes faded and is replaced by a negative force of energy, which causes a major imbalance. The treatment is designed to restore this balance. They are instructed to lie down with their arms stretched out to their sides. The shape of the patient's body should look like a cross. The curandero then brushes the body from head to toe with an herbal bundle using a plant called *pirul*. The brushing movements start from the chest down to the stomach and then to the legs and arms.

Before this treatment, the curandero sits with the patient and will discuss their troubles with them. The healer allows the patient to pour their heart out to them as they talk about their feelings about the trauma. While performing the brushing motion, the curandero recites a few prayers and then asks the patient to call for the lost spirit to come back to their body. Sometimes, the curandero's mouth is suddenly filled with a liquid that they spit out to wash the patient's face. When the spirit reunites with the body, the patient and curandero both feel it. The patient instantly changes as they recover and feel complete again, and the curandero senses their pulse returning to normal once more. Their body temperature also drops back to normal. In extreme cases of susto pasado, a curandero may conduct treatment for three whole days. During the treatment, the healer may ask the patient to drink from a prepared herbal drink, which has palm leaves floating on the surface.

With some pregnant women, the mother may transfer her fright to her unborn baby. To prevent this illness, a curandero instructs the mother to prepare a special drink. This is made by first heating some coals until red hot. Then the hot coals are dropped in a glass of warm water. The water is then sweetened with sugar, and then the mother drinks it immediately. Children are the most vulnerable to susto, and they usually appear pale, weak, and thin in stature as they rarely eat.

Another treatment for susto involves using a couple of branches from a sweet pepper tree and a candle. The candle is fixed on a small plate and laid on the floor. The child is then instructed to walk over the candle parting their legs on each side of the plate. The mother then takes the sweet pepper branches and brushes the child's body from head to toe and then from left to right, signaling the cross sign. A special prayer called credos is recited three times. The child is then left to rest with the two sweet pepper branches lying under his bed in a cross sign. After that, the mother walks away and calls her child's name, telling them to come to her and not be afraid anymore. This statement is mentioned three times as the mother leaves the room. The treatment should be repeated three days in a row at the exact time. It is believed that the child will be cured of susto by the third night.

There are many safe home remedies to try for various illnesses. Hot herbal teas can be used to drink or as a massage oil to treat many diseases. For example, cinnamon tea is excellent to soothe cold or flu symptoms. Cinnamon has anti-inflammatory effects, and it serves as an excellent method of aromatherapy as its smell spreads in the house, promoting relaxation. Chamomile teas are used to aid sleeping and prevent stress and anxiety. Mint tea is excellent for treating digestive aches and is wonderful at relieving migraines and headaches. It is refreshing aroma also helps in mild cases of asthma as it naturally causes muscle relaxation in the lungs helping with respiratory distress. Lemons and limes are used to treat coughs and colds as they are natural antioxidants. It can be mixed with honey to mask its bitter taste and to help soothe a rough cough.

Many curanderos are proficient in massage therapy or *sobadas*, which is prescribed for people who suffer from indigestion, muscle and joint pain, and even infertility. Massages are also used to help a person overcome emotional distress. Many modern-day curanderos and curanderas study to be chiropractors, which helps them to better understand the anatomy of the human body. Traditional massage therapies are used on patients when they have certain ailments as opposed to regular massages that are done mainly to promote relaxation. When a healer performs sobadas, they target the injured area in your body and do not massage the whole body as in a regular massage. The treatment may create discomfort and may even be painful depending on the severity of the injury. After treatment, the person is instructed not to shower to allow the maximum effect of treatment. The person is also told to stay warm to avoid getting a cold and asked not to eat before treatment or else they could feel nauseated due to the hard pressure.

Other therapies include a technique called smudging, which involves burning medicinal herbs around the sick person to cleanse their body. Typical herbs used in this treatment are sage and cedar. A special oil blend of eucalyptus, camphor oil, menthol, and turpentine oil is used to create a gel-like substance used as a medicinal rub to treat congestions, coughs, and other flu symptoms as it provides a warm sensation in the body.

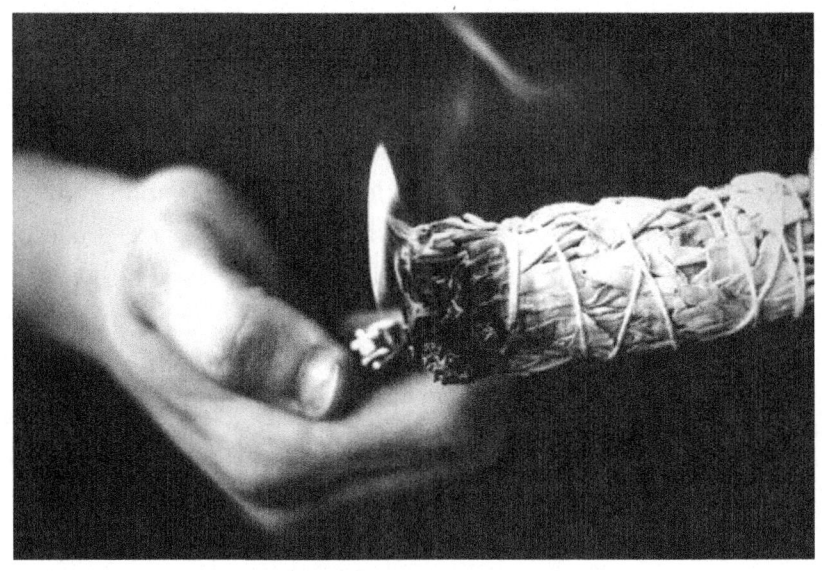

## Herbal Preparations

A curandero uses different herbs to make medicinal teas to drink, collects them in a bundle to brush on a patient's body, or combines them with oils to create topical medicinal pastes. Some herbs like Juniper are burnt as incense. Some are prepared by being mixed with alcohol to form a tincture, and yet others are prepared by mixing the herbs with water to form macerations. Herbs can also be made into ointments, pastes, and plasters like mustard plasters. Floral herbs like rosemary are combined with water to be used as a mouthwash.

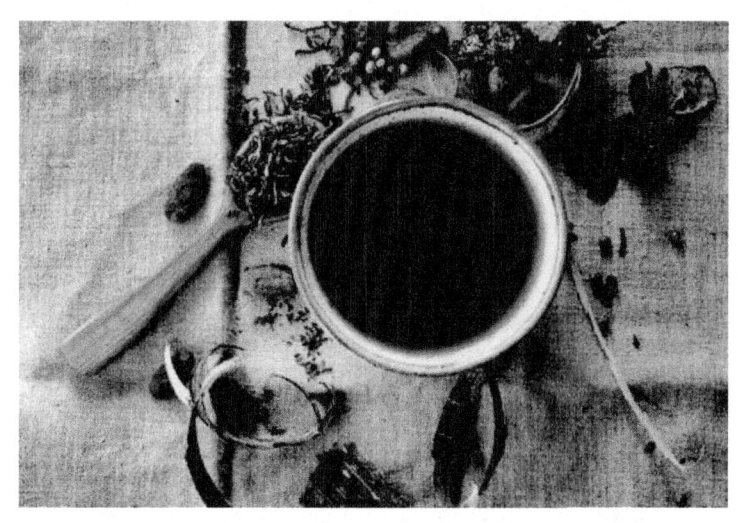

Some herbs are used to make medicinal tea by infusion - mixing the herbs with boiling water and letting it infuse for a while. Another type of preparation is called decoction, which involves adding the herb to the water and heating it at low heat without boiling until the water absorbs all the properties of the herb. The herb then is passed through a strainer leaving behind an herbal tea to drink. Macerations involve soaking herbs in water for a period no less than overnight, but they can be left for up to a week in water before being used. Tinctures are prepared by soaking mashed herbs in alcohol and storing the mash in a dark place for about a week. Then, it is taken out and strained before use. The best containers to use for all these preparations are glass containers to avoid any toxic reactions to the storage material that may affect the herbal concoctions or render them ineffective. It is best to dry the herbs before use, as their medicinal properties become more concentrated.

Bear in mind the potency of these preparations cannot be properly determined. Many factors affect the efficacy of plants - like their soil, environment, humidity, and size. If you're planning to use these homemade remedies, make sure to consult your doctor before trying out any preparations. We encourage you to do plenty of research before trying out any new herbs. You have to be careful not to add any poisonous parts to your tea. You have to learn about which plants can be boiled and which are to be consumed fresh because some plants become dangerous for consumption when exposed to heat.

You have to take care even if you purchase ready-made herbal preparations. A common remedy for empacho is called *greta,* which was found to include traces of lead monoxide, which is an extremely toxic compound. Some people use this treatment for ailments other than empacho like headaches. Prolonged use of lead monoxide may have devastating effects on your health as it may lead to blood poisoning or severe handicap.

In this chapter, we discussed various ailments which affect the body and how a Curanderismo healer treats each of these conditions. Don't attempt to perform these practices on your own. The procedures mentioned are carried out by experienced healers who have practiced Curanderismo for many years. You should not replace modern medicine with this traditional technique. You should consider it as a form of complementary medicine after asking your doctor. You need to do a lot of research before you choose the proper curandero or curandera to treat any ailments.

# Chapter 5: Limpia, or Spiritual Cleansing

Spiritual cleansing helps rid afflicted people of all negative energies and comes in various methods. However, these methods should only be used as a secondary option since you should see a doctor if you suspect you are suffering from a serious, possibly complicated medical issue.

This chapter begins by explaining what *limpia* is and how it can help people who are interested in trying it. We then go on to expand the different types of cleansing and items used in each therapy, such as a crucifix, herbs, citrus, fumigation, and egg cleansings.

## What Is Limpia?

Traditional healers are often consulted to perform rituals to heal both physical and spiritual ailments. In South and Central America, this practice is common since different types of diseases are viewed as impediments that lead to an imbalance between humans and their environment. Therefore, a traditional healer will seek to restore the balance between the individual and their environment as well as with the spiritual world. A limpia is often performed to cleanse individuals of negative energy, which is believed to cause some misfortunes.

A limpia is a spiritual practice commonly used to cleanse the body, soul, and mind of negativity. Limpias is used in different cultures, especially in Mexican curanderismo medicine. This is a beautiful process that involves the use of different elements such as flowers, plants, intentions, and prayers. Plant spirits and ancestors are used to heal spiritual and emotional imbalances that can be caused by trauma or acute shock. A cleansing ceremony will help support the emotional and spiritual body when it is undergoing challenges.

Limpias is also performed when a person is undergoing a major transition in life to help cleanse the mind and soul so that they can be focused on the goals they want to achieve. Many people believe that there are dark forces that can act as impediments and prevent them from achieving what they want to achieve in life. Spiritual cleansing ceremonies are known to remove blockages, bad luck, confusion, imbalances, witchcraft, bad karma, or end generational curses. Individuals suffering from unknown fears, addictions, and phobias can also get salvation from limpias.

The practice of limpia is believed to be very powerful in healing spiritual illness and helping solve physical health issues as well. However, you should know that this practice is not a replacement or substitute for medication. It is essential to visit a medical doctor when you are suffering from an illness that can be diagnosed and cured using modern medicines. Limpias provide spiritual healing, which may not be a remedy to all the health problems we may experience. Other illnesses are purely natural, and some are caused by accident, and such conditions require proper medication.

It is widely believed that a limpia brings protection, peace, clarity, rejuvenation and that it also opens up opportunities in life. It also helps you attract blessings and luck, which can go a long way toward turning your fortune around. If you are looking for a new job or want to try something different in life, it is possible to get blessings from a limpia.

# How Do You Know You May Need Limpia?

There are various signs to be considered to find out if a spiritual cleansing will be beneficial in your life. Relationship problems are common but, in some cases, they may be caused by elements such as bad luck. Traditionally, bad luck is widely viewed as a consequence of people's evil deeds. Therefore, if you have a good reason to believe that you were cursed by someone, you can seek spiritual intervention through the use of a limpia. The challenges you're facing may require a similar healing method if they are spiritual.

If you often feel weak, restless, and unable to cope with different things in life, you may also need a limpia. You can also consider the same solution if you suddenly have phobias or unknown fears impacting your life. Many people often fail to achieve their goals in life because of a fear-driven lack of confidence. You may also experience a constant unpleasant feeling that seems to affect everything you try. In most cases, the funny thing is that many people will not be aware of the source of their misery in life. This is when a cleansing therapy session comes in handy to clear your way so that you can pursue your goals with confidence.

Other signs that indicate you need a cleansing healing session include having a hard time and experiencing severe nightmares. Nightmares can lead to hallucinations, and your mind will not think clearly. All these issues can be traced back to evil spells that should be exorcised using spiritual cleansing.

If you get the feeling that someone is blocking you from moving forward, you will need some cleansing. Some people derive pleasure from the suffering of others. This is one of the reasons why some people will cast evil spells on other human beings. You can overcome this challenge by invoking a cleansing ceremony for guidance and protection from supernatural powers.

When performing a limpia, there are some tools you can use depending on your situation and the experience of the curandero.

Natural things are commonly used for spiritual cleansing ceremonies since they are believed to be pure. A spiritual healer conducting the ceremony will tell you the items required for a successful exercise. For instance, it is believed that a raw egg or other natural elements can absorb negativity because they are not tainted. If you do not want to call a spiritual leader, you can try the cleansing on your own. Whatever the case may be, there are certain things you will need to use to make the limpia effective. The following are some of the types of limpias you can perform when seeking spiritual guidance.

## Herb Cleansings

A ritual can be a quick fix, especially if you constantly feel off, lethargic, and uninspired. It will help you clear away the negative energy surrounding you. This can be alleviated by using herbal herbs cleansing to bring fresh and fantastic energy into your home and entire life. This practice is simple since all you need to do is to burn the preferred type of herbs recommended for your problems. When the smoke appears from the burning herbs, carry them around your home and walk with an intention in your mind. You need to be clear about what it is exactly that you want the burning herbs to help you with. However, if you are sensitive to smoke or have asthma, this type of ritual might not be ideal.

Before you start the ceremony, open the windows, and never leave the herbs burning unattended. The secret behind burning herbs is that they are believed to play a crucial role in absorbing all the negative energies that can be giving you problems in your body. In return, the burning herbs will provide positive energy, which encourages peace of mind. If you are cleansed, you can live in harmony with others and also overcome your fears.

People in different parts of the world burn various types of herbs to clear evil spells. For instance, burning cedar is often viewed as a great way to clear the air when you are experiencing bad juju. When you burn this type of plant, you will clear all the negative energy that may be lingering in your home. It also helps remove bad memories negatively affecting your life; remember that negative thoughts can affect the way you relate with others.

There are different types of herbs used in limpias, and the herbs used depend on the problem to be solved and geographic location. There is no one herb that can fix all problems, as each malady needs a specific herb for healing purposes. You can perform cleansing using bundles of fresh herbs tied together using a red or white string. The bundle should resemble a small hand-held broom, and it should be sprinkled with holy water. If you decide to do the ritual yourself, pray for the bundle, seeking guidance and restoration to normal health. To remove negativity, use the herbal broom to sweep your body in a downward direction. The herbal brooms can be from a combination of herbs or a single herb. As indicated above, your type of situation will determine the herbs you can use.

## Crucifix

Crucifix cleansing offers the benefit of creating a stronger connection with your spirit helpers. It is also used to break the dark work of spells, punish enemies as well as purge evil spirits and other demonic powers. The healer often administers this type of cleansing using a large hand-held crucifix. The crucifix is a very effective tool in the removal of the effects of any dark arts. Its effectiveness is significantly enhanced if it is made of metal or brass as opposed to plastic or wood.

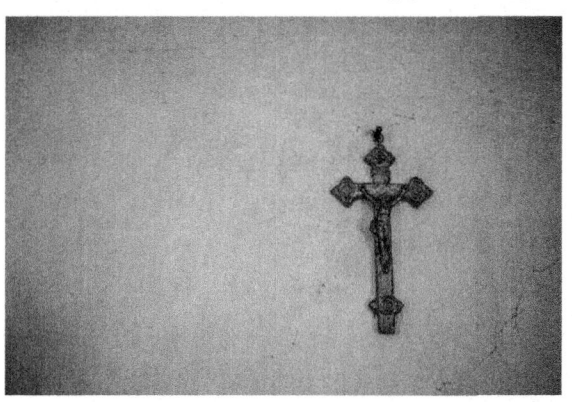

The healer will hold the cross and move it in small crosses around your body while reciting prayers. While this action is performed, you should also pray to ask for deliverance from whatever problem you are facing. The healer will repeat the motions; it is believed that crucifix cleansing draws negative energy from your body and surroundings. In turn, you gain positive energy, which rejuvenates your spirits. When you are feeling low, you need to find a way to lift your spirit, which is good for your mental and physical health.

## Citrus

Citrus cleansing is used to break stubborn energies that still linger after an attempt to remove phobias, nightmares, and mental disturbances. To perform this exercise, fresh uncut lemons or limes are used as they are most powerful for removing stubborn and other stagnant energies. These items can also act as a powerful defense against witchcraft. The good thing about using limes and lemons is that they possess powers that can break the effects of hexes, curses, and spells. You can dispose of the used citrus fruit using fire.

On a different note, the citrus diet can also play an equally similar role to cleansing. Citrus helps to detoxify your body and remove accumulated waste. The unwanted components sap your energy which makes you feel weak. Therefore, different types of citrus fruit (like limes, lemons, oranges, tangerines, and grapefruit) cleanse your body. You need to consult the doctor first before you begin your cleansing diet. The same applies to spiritual cleansing, which requires you to seek guidance from experts first before you do it.

From these two forms of citrus cleansing, it can be noted that they have a lot of things in common. Though nutritional cleansing is scientific, it is based on the same principles as limpia. According to empirical scientific studies, the accumulation of waste in the body affects its normal function. Consuming raw foods like citrus fruit can go a long way toward detoxifying the body while at the same time nourishing it. You can try citrus cleansing using your preferred method, as well as using the fruit of your choice.

# Fumigation

Fumigation is used specifically for soul loss activities. People who like to work with nature favor this method of cleansing since it provides the four elements of spirituality. First, you possess the energy of the plant and some elements of the earth. The second aspect is that you have the element of fire represented by the burning charcoal. The third aspect pertains to the element of air, which is smoke. Lastly, the spraying of holy water represents an element of water. In its natural form, water represents life.

When performing a spiritual cleansing, these four elements create a powerful combination that drives negativity out of your body. The body represents all components of the earth which include dust to dust and ashes to ashes which makes the process of spiritual fumigation appropriate for enhancing recovery from soul loss. If you are at a loss with your soul, you are likely to experience many challenges that can affect you spiritually. Other things like negative energy will also be prevalent and affect your wellbeing. The earth's components can go a long way toward helping you fumigate all the challenges you may be facing.

# Egg Cleansing

An egg is a crucial component of the womb since it bears new life. In the same vein, an egg can also be used to cleanse you of evil spells or negative energy to give you new life. This cleaning method involves rubbing the egg over your entire body, and you must pay special attention to the heart, head, stomach, hands, and feet. This form of limpia is multipurpose since it can be used to cure a variety of problems that include bad luck, spiritual and physical illnesses, stress, fatigue, nightmares, and hidden obstacles.

In its raw form, the egg is capable of absorbing things that don't belong to where they are found. For example, no one was born with bad luck, which means that it has no room in our lives. Therefore, the egg will remove any bad luck that must not be part of your life. Prayers play a part in the cleansing ritual, and the recipient's name is written on the egg. This will help create a link that will be used in the healing process. The healer may also write the name of the saint on the egg that will be used to heal a known physical problem. The egg is moved around the affected area while the healer is saying prayers.

The egg cleanse is known to help cure diseases like breast cancer. If you want to work on a specific problem, you call a specific Saint to aid you in the healing rite. If you are carrying strong and aggressive energy, the raw egg is said to explode when it comes into contact with you. During cleansing, it absorbs a lot of negativity, and this can cause it to explode when it is full of spiritual dirt.

If you are experiencing negative energy and other issues such as spells, bad luck, misfortunes, or anything else, you may need a limpia or spiritual cleansing. The prime purpose of spiritual cleansing is to get rid of any negativity that may be impacting your life and replace it with positive energy. As mentioned previously, different ailments or emotions will tell you what type of cleansing you need, and there are quite a few ceremonies that cover a lot of different situations from which you can choose. If you want to perform the exercise without a spiritual healer, make sure you have the right materials to use. Make sure you know what you will be doing.

# Chapter 6: Curanderismo and Eggs

Curanderismo relies on various tools, techniques, and ingredients to help patients who are suffering from any kind of problem. Whether it is a physical ailment, a spiritual problem, or a mental issue, there is a solution for it to be found in Curanderismo. Practitioners will use various things ranging from herbs to plants to animal fats and use these things in different ways to heal a malady. However, one of the most often used items for holistic healing is the humble chicken egg. Whether you are looking to relieve yourself of bodily pain, recover from burns or draw out negative energy, an egg can be helpful. In fact, eggs have even been used to predict the future, tell the gender of a child while it is still in the womb, and predict the occupation of a woman's future husband.

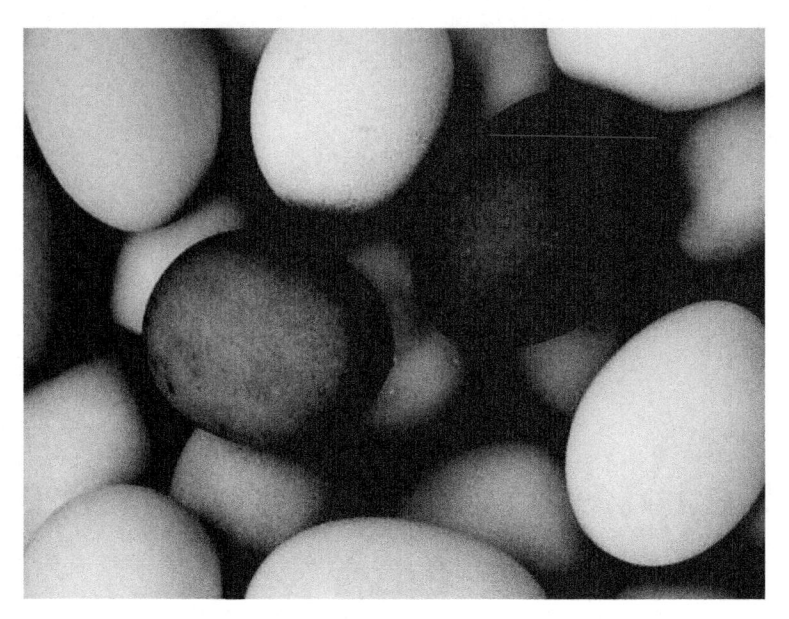

The use of eggs in traditional healing is something that is not only limited to South American culture but is something that is used in many different cultures across the world. All the way from South America to Europe, Rome, down to Southeast Asia, and even as far away as Far East Asia, egg treatments can be seen as a global phenomenon that has been used for thousands of years.

## Eggs and Healing

The process of cleansing or healing through the use of eggs in any form is known as *oomancy*. This is an ancient method of healing and has its roots in the old Roman and Greek traditions. In fact, "oo" is the Greek word for egg. Oomancy relates to a number of healing practices that are used to heal the body, mind, or spirit. Let's look at a few ways you can heal by using eggs.

One of the most common ways eggs are used to heal the body is to rub the egg on the body to bring down a fever. Whether this is a fever accompanied by a cold or just a fever on its own, this method fights all kinds of fevers equally well. All you need to do is get a clean egg and place it in a pot of water with some vinegar in it. Put this on the stove and bring it to a boil, letting it cook until the egg is well done and the yolk is nice and firm inside. This usually takes around ten minutes. Once the egg is done, take it out and cool it down under some tap water. The purpose is to bring the temperature down just enough so that you can handle the egg without burning your hands. Once the egg is at a comfortable warmth, hold it in your hand vertically so that you can roll the egg across the thickest part of your body.

You can start with your head and start rolling the egg across your forehead, down the sides of your face, down your neck, onto your shoulders, and then down your arms. When you reach your hands, you can loop the egg around your arm and also cover the inside of your arm, bringing it down to your torso, and then start rolling it downward. Continue as far as your waist, moving on to your thighs and shins. Also, for the legs, you can do it in two sections on each leg, with one round covering the outside of your legs and the second round covering the inside of your legs. In this way, you can go over your entire body and make sure you get every spot. Also, you can roll the egg around on your scalp and your face and cover your entire skull. You don't have to do this on your own. If you have someone who can help out, you can always get them to assist, especially when it comes to getting to hard-to-reach spots like your back. Once you have finished with the rubbing, you can throw the egg away. Also, you can use this remedy multiple times though most people will see a significant change in their fever after just a single use.

The next egg treatment is used to care for burns and bruises. This also involves rubbing an egg, but the process is slightly different. For this remedy, you need to boil the egg in plain water until it is well done. Once the egg is ready, you need to slice it open to remove the yolk. You are going to replace the yolk with a silver ring or a silver coin, or a similar-sized object made of silver. Then place the egg back together and tie it up in a piece of cloth or a small towel. Use this parcel and massage your injury with it, but there is no need to rub it all over the body. Keep the egg in the towel for a couple of days and use it to massage the injury frequently until the bruising or burn has healed completely.

## How to Do an Egg Cleansing

One of the more popular forms of treatment that eggs are used for is spiritual cleansing. This is a process known as limpia in Spanish. While the main purpose of the ritual is to cleanse the body, spirit, and mind, doing so also helps the person to improve their physical condition. In any case, when the person is having trouble with their body or their mind, it is the result of an imbalance in their energy - the harmony between body, mind, and spirit, or it is the result of negative energy. For instance, if a person has been to a place where they feel they have been surrounded by a lot of negative energy and they are feeling down because of that, the egg can help solve this problem. Similarly, if a person has been having trouble sleeping, experiencing bad dreams, or just been having unusual and uncomfortable thoughts, then a cleansing may be helpful.

In other cases, problems can have a very physical impact on the person. This is usually associated with the evil eye or with magic and spells. The evil eye is a very common problem that can be found in many cultures and traditions, and they all have their own way of dealing with it. What is more important is that the evil eye can affect a person in different ways. In some cases, it may have very physical consequences, such as the person getting sick, having trouble sleeping, eating, or being ill with any other kind of disease. In other situations, it can result in things like accidents and injuries or just unfold as a period of time during which the person starts experiencing bad luck and encounters a bad situation for no rational reason.

The evil eye is something that can be caused out of jealousy, envy, hatred, and any other kind of negative emotion passed on to you through the evil looks from someone who wishes you ill. Babies are particularly sensitive to the evil eye though it can affect elders just as much.

Some of the most common reasons people look into getting limpia done are:

- They are about to take on a major change in their life, such as getting married, starting a business, or moving to a new location.
- They are experiencing nightmares, strange accidents, insomnia
- They are experiencing sudden losses and tragedies for no reason
- Feelings of depression, lethargy, anxiety, or feeling mentally unwell
- Feeling like you have no options and are facing an obstacle in life

Limpia is something that you can perform on yourself on your own, or you can have an expert curandera help you through it. Moreover, you can also perform it on someone else who may need it, and it can also be used as a method of cleansing your home or other tangible assets you own.

To carry out an egg cleansing routine for yourself, you will need an egg, some salt, a white candle, and a glass of water. To get the best results, either use a fresh egg or take the egg out of the fridge a few hours before you plan to do the ritual. The same thing applies to the water. You need to have it at room temperature, so take it out of the fridge in good time. If either of the two things is too hot or too cold, the readings may change, and room temperature ingredients will yield the best results. If you have an altar in your home with a holy figure on it, you can place the egg and the water onto the altar near the holy figure to receive his/her blessings.

To prepare yourself for the ritual, it is always good to be clean. You can perform a spiritual bath, or you can just have a shower or bath as you normally would. To get the full feel of the experience, you can add some Epsom salts to your bath or use some nice aromatic bath soaps and salts.

If you are performing a spiritual bath, then you can sit in the bath for a few minutes - 15 minutes or so, and just talk to yourself and discuss all the things that are bothering you. State the intentions that you have for purifying yourself, cleansing yourself of negative energy, and washing away the toxins from the body. Once you have brought your mind, heart, and soul into the process, let the water calm you down and then wash yourself off, making sure that you also wash the tub out thoroughly and then have a quick shower to cleanse everything.

You can come out of the bath and also offer a small prayer and thank the deities you believe in. The prayer before the actual cleansing is a great way to focus your energy on the task ahead, and you can also take the egg and dip your hand into the water, holding the egg in your hand and praying with those items.

As you move onto the egg cleansing itself, you need to sit down somewhere comfortably, either on the floor or on a chair and light the candle. Let the candle burn all the way down without putting it out yourself. You can start to say a prayer if you are a Christian or may have a religious prayer you would like to use. If not, you can start talking to the universe and asking the universal energy to cleanse you of negative energy, thoughts, emotions, vibrations, and experiences.

Next, start with the egg on your head and just cup it gently in your hand, then rub it on your head and move onto other parts of your body ending with your feet. Ideally, the egg must come into contact with every inch of your skin, but you don't be too repetitive. You can redo some parts that you may think you have left out but generally try to get all areas covered in one or two passes at most. There are certain areas that you may not be able to reach, such as your back, and this is where you can have someone assist you in the process, or you can just try to reach these parts as much as you can, even if it doesn't come in direct contact with the egg.

If there are any areas where you are experiencing pain, maybe an injury, then make sure you get these areas and really focus your thoughts while you pass these regions. Christians who practice this form of cleansing will also start by making the sign of the cross with the egg and end by doing it again when reaching their feet. If you aren't religious, then pay attention to the beginning and end of the process and visualize positivity, and think positive thoughts.

After the cleansing, some people prefer to keep the egg as it is under their bed for a full day before they crack it open, while others prefer to just crack it open right away. In both cases, you crack it making sure it is at room temperature, into the same temperature water that you have waiting, and then look into what shapes the egg makes. If you are using two eggs, crack them into the same body of water.

If you plan to clean the house, start by opening all the windows to let the negative energy out of that space. Ideally, you should be alone in the house while you do it. If you live with family, ask them to go out for a few hours while you cleanse the home. Next, light the candle in a central part of the home. Take the egg, hold it in your hand, stretch your arm out in front of you, and start walking into each room and open area of the house. While you do this, recite a prayer, talk to the universe about positivity, and ask the universe to cleanse your home of negativity and evil. Once you have covered all areas of the house, you can break the egg into the glass of water, add salt to it, and flush it down the toilet.

## How to Read an Egg after Cleansing

When you have broken open the egg, the first thing that you look at is the yolk. In normal circumstances, the yolk will sink to the bottom of the glass. If the yolk remains suspended in the middle of the mixture or floats to the top, this is a bad sign. It means that someone is sending negativity and evil toward you, and you are suffering from a negative influence. Similarly, a broken yolk is not a good sign and means that someone is trying to harm you.

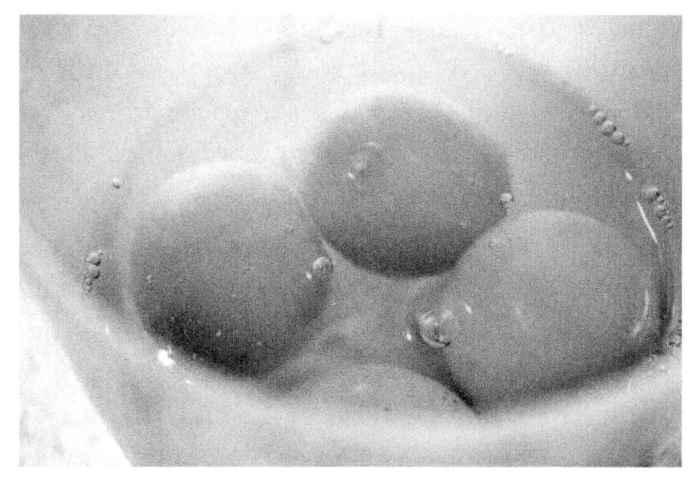

If the yolk has blood in it or spots in it, this could be a bad sign for your health and mean that you may face sickness.

If the liquid from the egg forms needles or spikes or sharp objects, this is not a good sign either; you should definitely consider doing more cleansings.

If you find two or more yolks in the glass, this could mean pregnancy, and it is usually seen as a sign of fertility and good news.

If the yolk appears nice and bright and the water is also clear, this is a great sign and means that your cleansings have either been successful or that there is nothing negative around you.

Similarly, suppose you see a lot of little bubbles around the yolk or on the surface or base of the water. In that case, this means that your ancestors, guides, teachers are watching over you and trying to absorb the negative energy that is coming your way.

Patterns or images such as flowers, the sun, or other things that are associated with positivity are always good signs.

Remember that cleansing is something you have to do on a frequent basis. If there is some kind of negativity in your life, and this shows up in your initial cleansing, then you have to perform more cleansings to solve these problems. The negativity that you see in the egg cleanse only indicates what could be happening in your life, so make sure you address these things with a doctor if it is a medical problem. Try to manage your relationships better if it is a social issue. Repeat the cleanse again to see your progress and make sure you are going in the right direction.

# Chapter 7: Mal De Ojo Healing

The evil eye superstition is one believed by many cultures and has its origins in the ancient times of most parts of the world. People believe the evil power of an envious eye can cause actual physical or mental illness. Many religions like Islam and Judaism acknowledge the evil eye, and holy verses of protection against it are included in both the Quran and Torah. From Greece and Turkey to Brazil and Latin American, many cultures believed that the eye possesses an evil force to be reckoned with. This chapter will discuss the history of *mal de ojo* or the evil eye, its negative effects, and how to protect against it.

## What Is Mal De Ojo?

Mal de ojo means "evil of the eye" in Spanish, and most cultures recognize the term as the "evil eye." People believe that negative or evil energy radiates from the eyes and is aimed at other people or things. Some cultures believe that the evil power of the eye is so apparent that you can sense its effects almost immediately.

It is believed that the origins of the evil eye date back thousands of years to the ancient Egyptian civilization. Other cultures then adopted this belief as it was transferred to the Greeks and ancient Romans. It is believed it was then carried to the lands that we know today as Spain more than two thousand years ago, and it was the Spanish who named it "mal de ojo."

Mal de ojo is perceived as a fake compliment of admiration to someone's possessions, physical beauty, or strength, or of their children. It is basically aimed at anything one person has that another doesn't and is the cause of great envy. When a person gives someone "ojo," it means they either intentionally or unintentionally give them an envious or jealous look. Latin cultures believe that the direct effect of receiving "ojo" causes an instant effect of heating the receiver's blood.

Some symptoms that result from mal de ojo include high fever, melancholy, loss of appetite, digestive issues, constant fatigue, insomnia, and drowsiness. People also believe that mal de ojo leads to misfortune, and many believe that all diseases are a result of some sort of evil energy cast on them through the evil eye. Suppose a person is involved in an accident, or their car breaks down, especially when it is usually kept in excellent shape, or any other freak accident happens out of nowhere. In that case, many believe that person is suffering from the result of the evil eye. After being afflicted with such accidents, many strong believers in the power of the evil eye will shout out, "I've been cast with the evil eye!"

While western medicine does not particularly acknowledge the power of the evil eye, many studies are concerned with medical conditions that may have been a direct result of the evil eye. These ailments can include anything from respiratory infections like severe pneumonia or bronchitis to the common cold, flu, and other viral or bacterial infections.

Some communities in Mexico believe that a child who passes a green stool, suffers from diarrhea, or has a physical abnormality such as one eye appearing smaller than the other are all signs that a powerful evil eye has afflicted the child.

# How to Protect against Mal De Ojo

Different cultures use various talismans to protect themselves from the mal de ojo. In Latin America, azabache stone (also known as "black amber") amulets and bracelets are worn daily as protection. People of the kabbalah faith wear a red string to divert the direction of the evil eye away from them. Arabs and Turkish people wear bracelets and necklaces with blue evil eye beads, and they sometimes hang amulets made up of these beads on any of their possessions, for example, cars, houses, and even their children's beds. Other amulets can be made from red and black beads and silver amulets with drawings of a blue eye in their pattern. Some cultures in Central America rub dried umbilical cords of newborn babies on eye sockets to cure a person of the effects of the evil eye.

Another common treatment involves rubbing an egg all over the person's body and then cracking it in a glass of water. The glass is then placed underneath their bed. This treatment is believed to absorb the evil energy of mal de ojo and protect against it. The shape formed by the egg as it hits the water is then thoroughly examined. If an eye shape or oval shape is formed in the yolk or egg white, it is an indication that the egg has absorbed the power of the evil eye. Some people believe that the egg shape gives an indication of whether the person with the evil eye is a man or a woman. The egg here represents birth and is often considered the sign of purity and innocence. The act of passing it over a person's body is believed to absorb all the evil spirits infecting the person. One of the most popular healing methods from the evil eye is the act of cleansing, which involves saying a few prayers while rubbing the egg all over the person's body.

A variation of this treatment includes using a raw egg to encircle the air above an afflicted person's head. The egg is then placed in a bowl underneath that person's pillow overnight. In the morning, the egg is checked to see if it is still raw or was cooked through the night. A cooked egg is an indication of being cursed with mal de ojo because of the heated blood. Many people refer to curandera to help them get rid of the evil eye. Christians may also refer to priests to be anointed with oils and holy water to get rid of evil spirits.

In ancient times, people wore bronze amulets and sometimes cowbells to fight evil spirits caused by mal de ojo. Some people use phrases like "May God bless you and protect you from the evil eye" because they believe that blessing someone with the power of God will protect them from the evil spirits of mal de ojo. Religious parents widely use this practice as they bid farewell to their children when they leave the house or go on a long trip.

Some cultures use hand gestures to protect against the evil eye. Italians use a fig gesture by imitating its shape with their fist or a horned sign with their hand to protect against the evil eye. In the Caribbean, the gesture of extending the index finger is believed to have a protective effect by diverting the direction of the evil eye. A person would point their index finger toward the person they feel is giving them ojo. In many Middle Eastern cultures, people extend their palm in front of the face of a person who is directing the evil eye at them. This simulates the hamsa or khamsa hand amulet, an open hand sign usually blue in color. Many cultures, such as the Turkish, Arab, Trinidadians, and Tobagoans, believe the color blue is guaranteed to divert the powers of the evil eye.

Each country or region has its own ways of protecting against the evil eye. Some people use potions and charms like amulets or bracelets, while others use garlic to steer the evil eye away from a person.

Some Mexican cultures use red strings tied around children and babies' right wrists. The children continue to wear the string until they are old enough to conduct clear speech so that they are able to say prayers to cast off the evil spirits of mal de ojo. Other regions may attach a small amulet that resembles the eye of a deer, which is called "*ojo de venado*," which is thought to have protective effects against the evil eye. The ojo de venado comes from the seed of a Mucuna shrub.

Caribbean cultures believe a pinch in the arm is sufficient to divert the power of the evil eye, as long as it is done at the same moment the evil is cast. For example, when a person is giving you a compliment or you feel them giving you a prolonged gaze, you should pinch your arm to reverse any negative energy radiating from their gaze. Other people believe that swimming in the sea is sufficient to avert the evil eye.

Indian cultures have a tradition of drawing a black dot on a baby's forehead to divert the glance of the evil eye. They also practice a ritual where they create a broom made from palm leaves or use peacock feathers to brush over a person's whole body. This ritual is used to get rid of any sickness caused by the evil eye and is targeted at specific areas in the body.

The Greeks have many testing methods for the presence of evil spirits caused by the evil eye. People refer to their local healers who recite a few prayers passed down through oral tradition from their ancestors, specifically from a person of the opposite gender. These prayers are believed to avert the evil eye. They also believe that when a person starts to yawn during this treatment, it means that person is afflicted. The healer may also yawn several times while reciting their prayers. Another method to indicate the presence of the evil eye is by dropping a drop of oil in a glass of water to see if it floats, which it will under normal conditions. However, if the drop of oil sinks to the bottom, that is an indication that an evil eye has been cast on that person. Another version of the oil test is to add a couple of drops of oil and watch to see if they touch each other and merge, which also means there is an evil eye involved.

Another method of testing is piercing a few cloves with a pin. These cloves are then held with a pair of scissors over a lit candle. The healer uses the pierced cloves to make the sign of the cross over the person who is believed to have been cast with the evil eye. If the evil eye is present, the pierced cloves will burn quietly or explode. The healer then asks the patient who they were thinking about during the session. The person who came to mind is thought to be the one who casts the evil eye. This test aims to find out who cast the evil eye so that the patient is more careful around them or never invites them into their house. The person may also choose to wear a protective blue bead as a precaution.

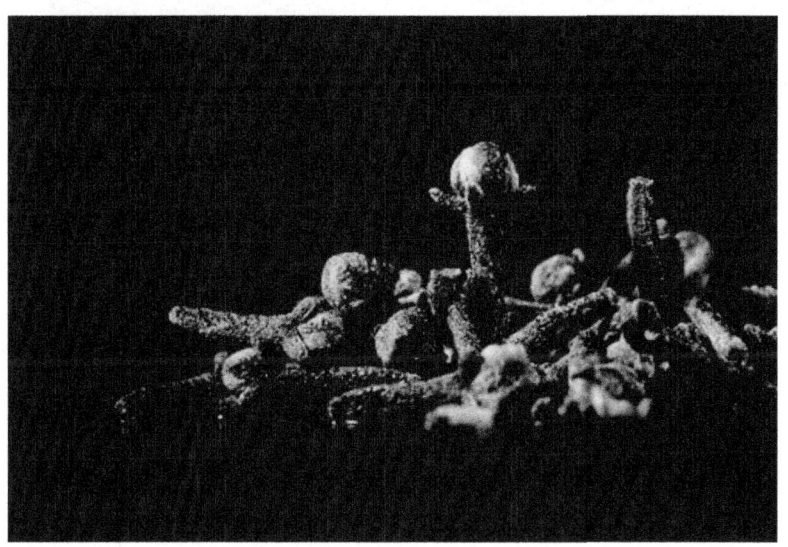

The pin piercing method is similar to that practiced in modern-day Egypt and dates back to hundreds of years, where a human-shaped paper cut-out called "*aroosa*" or doll is used in the ritual. A pin is used to pierce the head part of the paper where the eyes lie. The person performing this practice will say a few words, including the names of people they want protection from while piercing the paper doll's eyes with a pin. This practice can be done for anyone and by anyone and is believed to be a precautionary measure to protect against the evil eye.

## Who Are Most Vulnerable to Mal de Ojo?

Children, especially newborns, are believed to be the most vulnerable to mal de ojo. They are the most susceptible to deep stares from people who can accidentally give them the ojo when they are admiring their angelic appearance and captivating looks. It is believed that a single mal de ojo can make a child extremely sick. Pregnant women, as well as beautiful and physically strong or fit people, are also susceptible to mal de ojo.

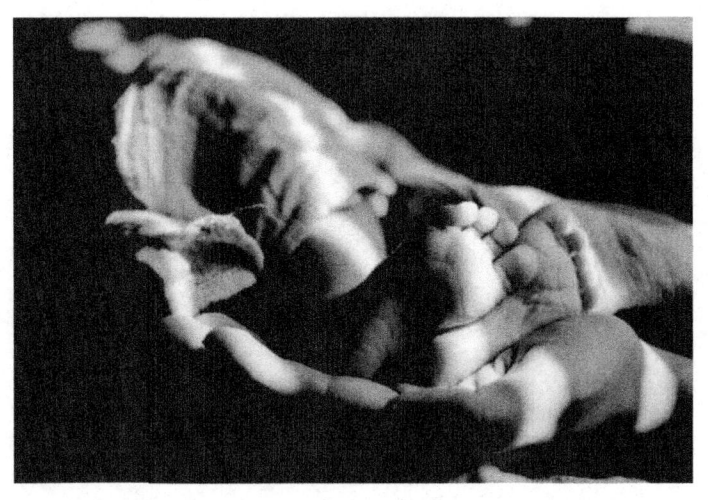

Some people in Caribbean communities also believe people can direct evil energy when they pat a child on the head or stare at them and admire them for too long. Parents can even do this, especially those who are obsessed with their babies or children. Other members of the family can also unintentionally afflict a newborn with the evil eye. This is why most parents make bracelets out of jet beads to be given to their newly born babies as a precaution because it is normal for all family members to express their admiration for newborns, which many cultures believe is one of the sources of the evil eye.

What makes people vulnerable to mal de ojo is that they sometimes get ojo from people they least suspect. They may receive an admiring gaze from someone who has just a glimmer of envy or jealousy, which is sometimes more than enough to affect the person with evil energy.

Some cultures frown upon public admiration of a newborn, like in India and Greece. This is because people believe that giving too many compliments in public will draw the powers of the evil eye. Some parents believe that to reverse the effect of the evil eye after praising a child calls for spitting in their face to make them appear imperfect so that the evil eye will not fall on them any longer. Muslims have a habit of saying "Mashallah" after giving any compliment. This phrase means "what God willed," which is used to bless and protect a person or a child from the evil eye.

## Curanderismo Treatments for Mal De Ojo

Using the egg cracking treatment, a curandero will examine the egg's shape to determine whether a person has been afflicted by the evil eye. If that turns out to be the case, the curandero uses special medicinal plants to cleanse the negative aura or air around the person afflicted by the evil eye. These plants usually include basil and a herbal blend that may include marijuana leaves and alcohol, which is added into a tub of warm water. The patient is then instructed to bathe in this water. These ancient cures have been practiced for many years and have been proven effective in Latin American cultures.

The curandero may also use a massaging technique to divert evil energy away from the person's body. They usually chant a few prayers as the whole treatment seems to be a ceremonial ritual.

It is important to note that not all people who give the evil eye are bad people. It is just possible that when you admire something for a long time, you could start developing feelings of jealousy and envy, emotions that carry negative undertones, and thus negative energy.

This is interpreted as the evil eye in many cultures and religions, and each one has different and unique ways of averting these evil spirits.

This chapter discussed the definition of the evil eye (or mal de ojo) and its meaning in different cultures. We explored how its history dates back to the ancient Egyptians and how each culture uses different types of talismans and amulets to protect themselves and their loved ones from the negative effects of the evil eye.

# Chapter 8: Susto Healing — Retrieving Lost Souls

This chapter focuses on "susto," also known as "soul loss" or "shock." It starts by explaining the concept's meaning, implications, symptoms, and causes. Susto is often confused with other forms of mental illnesses, and recommendations are provided for the measures you should take. The last part of the chapter describes in detail how a curanderismo ritual for cleansing this type of sickness is performed.

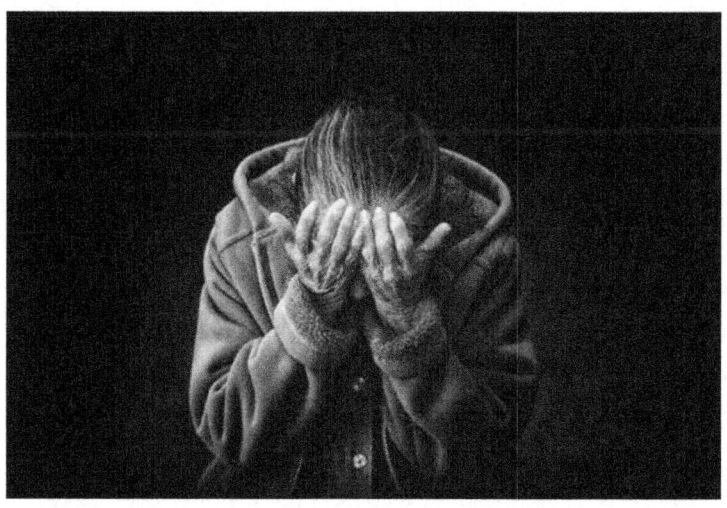

# What Is Susto?

*Susto* is a condition that causes intense emotion often felt when one experiences a sudden shock or traumatic event like the loss of a child or a car accident. This is also known as "soul loss," "shock," or "loss of the shadow." Traditionally, it is believed that when you experience soul loss, the soul will leave your physical body, and it will encounter challenges to find its way back.

# Susto and Culture

Susto is widely viewed as a syndrome that is culture-specific, and it reflects the belief system of a specific group. For instance, people of Mexican descent believe that soul loss is caused by factors like family fights, the spirits of the deceased, and the use of drugs. As you are going to see below, diarrhea, vomiting, and cold sweats are some of the symptoms associated with this particular condition.

Susto is a form of cultural illness common among Latin American cultures. Susto is viewed as a culture-bound syndrome. These syndromes often have a significant impact on behavior and cause substantial effects on the lives of the afflicted person and those of their family and friends. Though some people often confuse it with mental illness, soul loss is viewed as a syndrome rather than a sickness. A syndrome is defined as a group of symptoms representing a certain disease or disorder characteristics.

Different syndromes usually work together, and the pattern of symptoms produced can indicate a specific social condition that affects the people within a recognized ethnic group. Some of the syndromes can be culture-bound, like Anorexia Nervosa, while others are biological syndromes such as Down's syndrome. In medical anthropology, the culture-bound syndrome is described as a combination of somatic and psychiatric symptoms that are viewed as an identifiable disease peculiar to a specific culture or society.

However, the disease does not make any changes in the structure or biochemical functions of the body organs. Furthermore, the condition cannot be recognized in other cultures. Some mental disorders are conditioned by the cultures in which they are found. For instance, susto is more prevalent, especially in Latin America, and is also widespread in Mexico. From a personalistic medical systems perspective, loss, damage, or spirit possession are believed to be caused by supernatural beings. In some cases, they may be caused by people or unpleasant social situations, as already indicated above.

Since susto is associated with a specific culture, this means that a group of people will share the same view. However, the notion of culture-bound syndromes is still controversial as many doctors, anthropologists, and psychologists reject it. For example, Western Traditional Medicine does not recognize this kind of illness. They associate it and lump it in with anxiety disorders.

## Causes of Susto

The advocates of susto believe that soul loss has different destabilizing effects on different individuals. It is a condition caused by various influences, and the things that are perceived as frightening to one individual may not be scary to another. However, the bottom line is that susto is usually caused by a traumatic experience or anything that can lead to physiological pain. The condition is more common in women though it can also be found in children and men.

Several incidents can cause susto like the unexpected death of a child or close loved one. Many parents find it extremely difficult to accept this kind of loss, and this can severely impact their mental health. Most people feel as if they may as well be dead following the untimely death of a loved one. These extreme emotions cause the soul to temporarily leave the body, which is why some special form of healing is required to take account of the absent soul.

The sudden or unexpected noise from a barking dog or any other deafening sound can have a lasting impact on some people, while others are completely unaffected. If one is exceedingly terrified, one can experience behavior-altering shock. Accidents are also common factors that can lead to susto. They can include car collisions, falling from a horse, or tripping over something. The incident can stay in your mind for a long period, causing sustained nervousness.

If you share a hospital ward with someone who later dies, you could be severely affected by the incident. And this is likely to cause mental instability, which affects the mind. Another traumatic event includes an encounter with a ghost. This will give you nightmares and make it difficult for your spirit to find its way back to your body. If you are forced to do something against your wishes, you can also experience susto. Furthermore, you can find yourself experiencing soul loss if you are in a situation that makes you angry. Anger is the worst enemy and can destroy you if you fail to control it.

## Common Symptoms of Susto

The symptoms of susto are wide and varied since people are different. Some of the common signs of this condition are restlessness during sleep or feeling weak on waking up each morning. During the day, you will feel drowsy and tired. As a result, you may end up failing to do anything productive. Individuals suffering from this kind of illness can also experience a lack of appetite together with a loss of interest in taking care of themselves. In other words, you lack focus on anything, and you cannot make a distinction between good and bad.

Individuals suffering from susto often experience becoming irritated irrationally quickly and are easily started by minor things. Heart palpitations are also characteristic of people with this condition. All these signs indicate that your heart and mind are unsettled, which leads to fear of the unknown. You can also experience anxiety or general fear that something could happen to you. When you live in constant fear, you find it hard to concentrate on productive things, which impacts everything you do.

Other signs that you may be suffering from susto include nervousness and unexplained sadness. You don't know why you are sad or feeling nervous even while you may be living in a safe and comfortable place. Constant crying among children is another symptom of this condition. Many people believe that supernatural powers cause these symptoms and that the condition requires spiritual remedies.

## How Might Susto be Confused with Other Mental Illnesses?

The above symptoms are often confused with other types of mental illnesses. For instance, western-trained medical professionals associate these symptoms with clinical depression or excessive emotional stress. These are viewed as mentally related illnesses that many different life events can cause. If you fail to achieve your personal goals, you are likely to experience stress and depression. Many other factors cause conditions like anxiety or insomnia. Therefore, it is a good idea to visit a professional medical practitioner who will diagnose your condition to see if it is related to mental illness.

In some instances, it is difficult to differentiate between susto and mental illness as defined by western medical professionals. According to the advocates of susto, different stress factors can influence the bio-psychological structure of a human being. Socio-economic factors are also to be taken into account when making a diagnosis. Poverty and social class have a significant influence on stress factors. While susto is described as a Culture-bound Syndrome, it displays symptoms consistent with depression, anxiety, and post-traumatic stress disorder. Therefore, you should try to verify the exact condition you may be suffering from before you seek treatment.

### Healing the Spirit

Different methods can be used to heal susto, like taking herbs, praying, visiting a curandero, talking to a psychologist, or drinking holy water mixed with herbs. Various groups of people view susto treatments from different perspectives. Other people, particularly Mexicans, believe that the condition can self-heal, while even more believe that one can prevent it by staying calm and, in most cases, that emotionally strong and young people are less vulnerable. The other issue that can complicate the treatment of susto is that it is viewed from different perspectives based on where you live and whose advice you seek. Some people are of the view that your beliefs can change once you get into contact with other cultures. Therefore, you should choose the most appropriate healing method that is in harmony with your own belief system.

### Medication

If you visit a medical doctor, you are likely to be diagnosed with depression, and you will get a prescription for antidepressant pharmaceuticals. In curanderismo, susto can be treated with herbal remedies or ritual cleansings, which will restore your body's balance, and your soul will be able to return unhindered. There are different types of medicines you can take orally to cure mild cases of susto. For instance, you can take tea infused with marijuana, brazilwood, or orange blossoms. This type of treatment is natural, and it helps cure symptoms like insomnia, nervousness, despondency, anorexia, listlessness, diarrhea, and involuntary muscle tics. The good thing about natural remedies is that they have no side effects like other modern treatments.

## Perform Curandero Rituals

Another effective treatment for susto involves different rituals that are performed by a healer. If the ritual is practiced soon after the occurrence of the traumatic event, the results are likely to be better. It is essential to remember the event and not try to suppress it. Traditionally, a curandero performs the ritual to cure susto.

The ceremony can involve lengthy performances of ritual actions, which can also involve the patient's relatives and friends. Each session begins with prayers that are directed to the Catholic saint of the village. After the prayers, special herbs and a chicken egg are moved over the patient's body to absorb negativity and illness. The egg can be left in the position where the soul loss has occurred. Gifts are also used to appease the supernatural being with the patient's soul.

Part of the exercise includes partially stripping the patient who is shocked by liquor that is released from the curandero's mouth. Massage is another activity performed on the patient. The patient is also put on a bed near a hot stove and covered with warm blankets to encourage sweating, which is part of the treatment process. In different places, similar methods are used to treat susto, and a curandero conducts the ceremony. The ceremony is also called barrida or "sweeping," which refers to a fresh bundle of herbs that is used to sweep over the patient's body to get rid of negative forces.

Other curandero rituals are specifically meant to heal on psychological or spiritual levels. Certain curses can only be cured using specific treatments. For instance, the evil eye is a curse that comes from a malevolent look. This condition can be treated with spiritual cleansing. As indicated, the ceremony requires some rosemary plants and a chicken egg. After rubbing the egg over the body, the curandero breaks it into a glass and examines the pattern it creates in the water. The curandero will base their predictions on the shapes they observe or see in the glass, and this will determine the course of action they should take when healing the patient.

There are different types of susto, and some are mild while others are complicated. In western medication, symptoms are used to diagnose the problem. However, curanderismo diagnoses the problem according to the individual. The curandera will take into account your personality, mode of thinking, experiences, patterns of life, fear, and the event they feel is the cause of the problem. Since there are many causes of susto, the curandera needs to know the exact thing that drives you to visit them. They will use all this information to determine how they will deal with your particular case.

A simple spiritual ceremony is conducted for a mild susto, as shown above. However, if the case is complicated, the curandera will lead the proceedings with the help of an assistant. All ceremonies are accompanied by prayers, and this is where an assistant comes in handy. Before the beginning of the ceremony, the healer selects a certain area on the floor and sprays holy water there to cleanse it. The holy water is also used in the ritual to bring blessings to the afflicted patient.

The curandera asks the patient to lie on the floor and stretch their arms out while keeping their feet together in such a way that a "cross" is formed by the body. Four white candles are first blessed, then lit, and one each is placed near the head, feet, and each hand. The patient is asked to remain in the same position while praying silently for the return of the soul. The curandera creates an herbal broom using fresh twigs of basil, rosemary, and rue. The twigs are tied with a red string to form a handheld broom.

When the broom is ready, the assistant then lights copal incense which they hold while walking around the patient and making crosses with the smoke produced. At the same time, the assistant will be reciting some prayers. The curandera sweeps the patient's body using a bundle of herbs and calls the soul to return. The ceremony usually takes about an hour, and when it comes to an end, everyone is extremely tired. The curandera then asks the patient to sit and sip some fresh tea brewed from mint.

The ceremony will be performed for three consecutive days, and the curandera calls the spirit in a louder and more forceful way. Many people prefer to hold the last activity of the ceremony on a Friday since it is a powerful day. The patient will be healed by the third day. The ritual is closed with prayers, and the curandera sprays perfume over the patient.

Susto is a form of illness that causes intense emotion, which is often felt when one experiences a sudden shock or a traumatic event like the loss of a child or a car accident. It is also known as "soul loss" or "shock." Different signs can help you determine if you are suffering from susto. It is essential to consult a medical doctor first since the condition usually resembles other forms of mental illnesses in the western medical world. To cure this condition, different methods can be used depending on your situation.

# Chapter 9: Day-to-Day Curanderismo

As wonderful as the practice of curanderos is, curanderas practitioners have been dwindling in numbers. This is mainly due to a severe lack of proper and up-to-date resources on the discipline. Unless you are getting your knowledge from a trusted book or a practicing healer, it is quite difficult to find not just information but authentic information. Why is that?

Several curanderismo alternative medicine practices have been appropriated by people looking to make easy money from tourists looking for a "psychedelic experience." However, what's more distressing is that holistic practices like curanderismo are now becoming a trend, often practiced for prestige, profit, or aesthetics rather than for the authentic and original healing it can offer. The truth is, curanderismo is rooted in ancient traditions that were developed and practiced in the lands of Latin America using native plants and herbs.

It is a holy practice with a cultural significance that the practitioner must be aware of and respectful toward. More importantly, as you start incorporating curanderismo in your day-to-day, modern life, you need to stay true to the roots as much as you can. Ultimately, the practice is not just about the rituals or the plants, but it is about thoughts, intentions, and the bond between a practitioner and the life around them, through which they acquire their ingredients.

This chapter will show you all the ways you can incorporate curanderismo in your daily life and how you can apply what you've learned in the previous chapters.

## Ingredients to Keep Handy

Eggs: Used for spiritual cleansing and healing bruises, burns, and fever, eggs can come in handy quite a lot, so be sure to keep some around.

### Rue/Rosemary Water

Rue water is relatively easy to make, and it is quite a beneficial mixture to have because of its ability to cleanse negative energy.

You will probably find that you have the ingredients you need for this practice in your kitchen, so it is not difficult to start your own healing therapy.

### You'll Need:

- 1 Fermentation crock
- 1 Gallon of rainwater or purified water
- 1 Cup of fresh rosemary or rue leaves
- 1 Cheesecloth
- 1 thin rope

Now you have your ingredients together, you can create your own rue water.

### Instructions

1. Pour the purified water into the crock, then drop the rosemary or rue leaves on top.

2. Cover the top area with the cheesecloth and tie it with the rope.

3. Make sure that you've secured the crock tightly with the rope or a rubber band to avoid any kind of leakage, then leave your rue water in an area where the moonlight can reach it.

4. Let it sit there for an entire moon cycle, and make sure you bless the water once you place it in the moonlight.

5. After it completes its moon cycle, drain the water into smaller jars and store them in a cool and dark area.

You can now use your rue water to spiritually cleanse your altar.

If instead of rue, your herb of choice is rosemary, you can go ahead and replace one for the other while following the same recipe.

## Agua Florida

Also known as Florida water, agua Florida is an alcohol-based mixture used to clear out heavy negative energy and spiritually cleanse a space. It is always a good idea to keep some around for when you may need it.

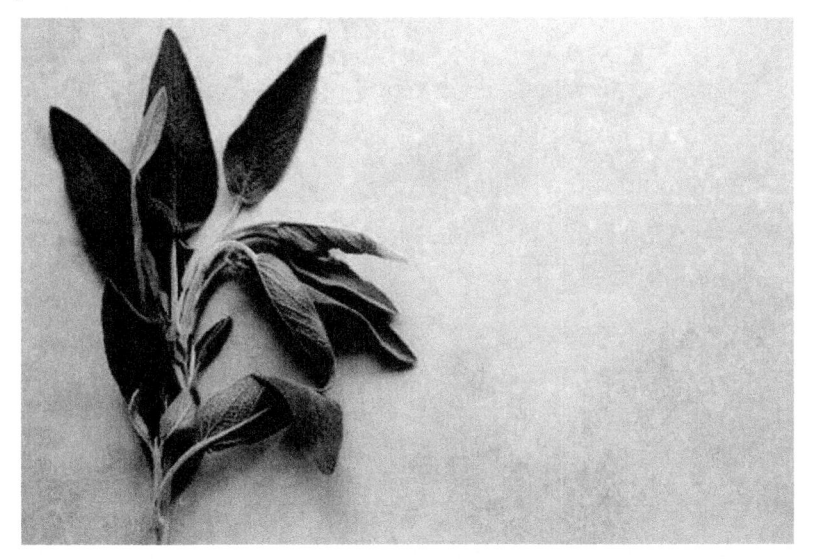

You can either buy your agua Florida or make it. Neither is a better option than the other, but you may find that, over time, you'll come to prefer homemade agua Florida to the store-bought alternative. Seasoned curanderos prefer putting specific intentions in their herbs, plants, and mixtures, so they try to grow/make what they can.

**You'll Need:**

- 6 Cups of Vodka
- 1/2 Cup dried sage
- 1/2 Cup dried lavender
- 1/2 Cup dried cedar
- ½ Cup Dried Sweetgrass
- A Cheesecloth

- 2 Clean glass jars for preparation and storage

**Instructions**

1. It is a simple recipe to follow. What you need to do is put your herbs, along with the vodka, in one jar and let them infuse for two weeks.

2. You can also place your jars under the moonlight to allow the mixture to capture the moon's positive energy.

3. After two weeks, use a cheesecloth to strain out the liquid into the second jar.

4. Close the lid, then store the agua Florida, and use it when needed.

Frankincense

You may recognize the name from the Bible's description of the interaction between the three wise men and newborn Jesus. In curanderismo, Frankincense is known for its multiple health benefits and positive spiritual effects.

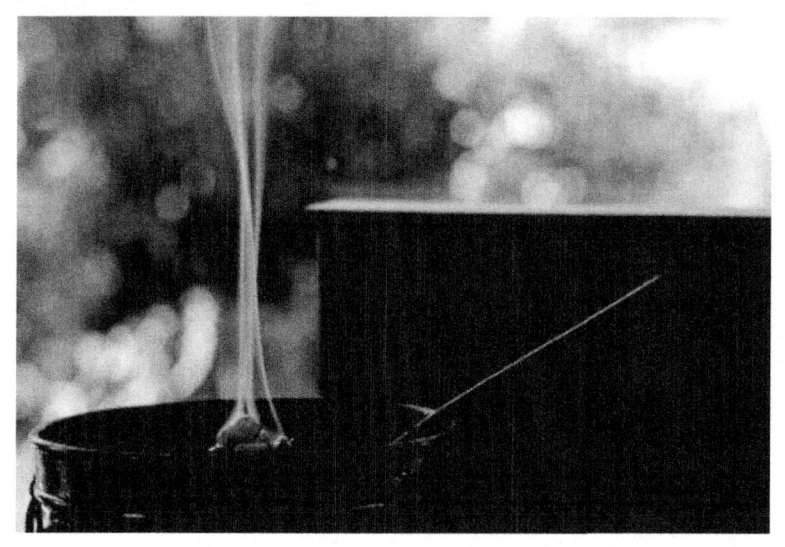

Frankincense oil is a scientifically-proven antimicrobial and antibacterial. In addition, it has been shown to have antidepressant qualities. Spiritually, it helps calm one's spirit and space, allowing people to better connect and get in touch with their whole being: mind, body, and soul.

**You'll Need:**

- Carrier Oil
- Frankincense oil

**Instructions**

1. To use the oil, mix it with a carrier oil; sweet almond, coconut, or jojoba.

2. Dilute it, then apply it to your body.

3. You can also add the mixture to a diffuser over a candle. The flame will do the work for you, spreading frankincense vapors through the air.

**Lemons**

Yet another household item that is capable of absorbing negative energy is the humble lemon. Although, two of its more popular uses are as an antibacterial and an aid to digestion.

Lemons are acidic, which means:

1. Lemons and their juices create an inhospitable environment for bacteria.

2. The acid in the lemons breaks down food in the stomach, facilitating digestion.

**Herb Bundle**

There is absolutely no limit to the number of herbs you can add to your bundle, but you must have one. Herbs are imbued with loads of benefits that help the whole patient; mentally, emotionally, and spiritually. Using a bundle allows you to get the most out of all your herbs.

The great idea is to create several bundles, each charged with a specific intention and dedicated to a specific purpose.

Some of the herbs you can use are:

- Rosemary
- Rue
- Tobacco
- Lavender
- Sage
- Mint
- Pepper Tree
- Basil

These herbs can then be tied up in a bundle and brushed over a space or one's body for purification purposes.

Once again, keep in mind that your intentions go a long way toward reinforcing the power of the ritual. When you're preparing your herbs and mixtures, make sure you show gratitude to your ingredients while focusing your thoughts on what you hope to get out of them.

## Amulets

These are a great way to carry your beliefs with you in your day-to-day life, as a constant reminder that the power is with you. When times get hard, you can always look to them for support, especially when you feel like you need something to get you through the day and remind you of what truly matters.

## Milagros

Milagros, also known as "miracles," are small metal charms fashioned in the shape of symbols, animals, saints, elements of nature, and some other forms. Initially, milagros were used as tokens to repay saints after receiving a favor.

People would ask a favor from a saint of their choice. Then, after they've received what they asked for, they would visit the saint's shrine and offer their milagro along with a prayer of thanks.

Ancient Curandero/as, specifically, channel their intentions into milagros or bless the small charms. They then give them to their patients so they benefit from the milagro's energy and benefits - which could range from good fortune to curing a physical ailment to protection against negative influences.

Milagro designs work on three levels being physically, mentally, and spiritually. For example, charms in the shape of a head could be used to bring about some mental or spiritual clarity, but they can also be used to cure headaches.

Specific milagros and their meanings:

- **Dog:** Dogs are known for their loyalty, but they are also known for their ability to watch over sheep herds. Dog milagros are commonly used for protection, guidance, and safety.

- **Heart:** The heart could be taken to refer to heart conditions. At the same time, it could also refer to romantic relationships or something to do with your emotional wellbeing.

- **House:** This could mean the actual house, the people living in it (family and loved ones), or a place/person whom you consider to be your home. It is a common milagro carried by those who travel a lot to keep them connected to their loved ones back home.

- **Body Parts:** As you may have guessed, body part milagros can be used to heal or protect a specific part of one's body.

The beauty of curanderismo seen here lies in the fact that the symbols are always open to interpretation. Keep in mind that symbols are a tool used to focus intentions and thoughts or invoke a saint's presence. It is never about the symbol itself as much as it is about the intentions behind carrying the symbol.

**Piedra de Iman**

Commonly known as lodestone, *piedra de iman* is made of a mineral called magnetite. As you may have guessed from the name, this type of stone is naturally magnetized.

In rituals, this stone can be used to attract opportunities and good fortune, thus bringing you closer to your goals; professional, personal, or otherwise.

The stone can also be carried around to attract such things and to help keep you stay grounded and balanced throughout the day.

### Beads

Beads are a big part of several religions and cultures, like Christianity, Buddhism, Hinduism, and Islam. In curanderismo, they play a big role when it comes to focusing one's intentions on a specific prayer. Through using beads and reciting prayers, one can also channel positive energy into the beads, thus blessing them.

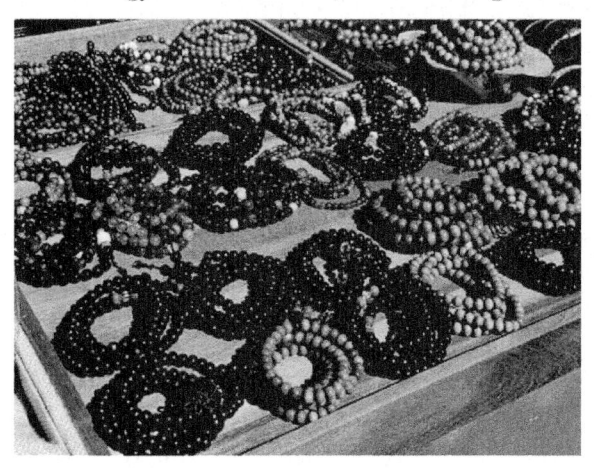

### Horseshoes

They are commonly known for being a lucky charm, but did you know it all started with ancient practices like curanderismo? Horseshoes are believed to attract good luck and success while warding off evil or bad luck. Although, the effects depend on the intentions of the horseshoe's wearer, and in some cases, its makers.

A great tip to boost the effects of your horseshoe amulet is to spray it with agua Florida or rue water.

### Prayers

A common mistake that is often made is thinking that some prayers work "better" than others. Prayer is not a well-constructed paragraph that one memorizes and uses whenever they please. Prayer is a group of words spoken, thought, or meditated on which come from the heart and with serious intention.

The beauty of prayer is that you needn't be somewhere specific or doing a particular ritual to pray. You can pray for guidance before going into a job interview or when you're facing a challenging decision. You can also pray for healing when you're sick. You can pray when you want to give thanks to your spirit guides, angels, or saints.

Prayer is a gateway and a form of communication between humans and higher beings, and so, if you treat it with the reverence it deserves, you'll make the most out of it. Prayers can also be used to bless amulets, mixtures, herbs, food, spaces, altars, and everything in between.

## Altars

Your altar is your sacred space where you get in touch with the spiritual, be it your own spirit, the spirits of your ancestors, your spirit guides, or saints. Altars are also supposed to be a calm and safe space that allows you to focus and connect. Needless to say, altars are very personal because the ties each individual has to the spiritual realm are unique to them.

### Creating Your Altar

We all have specific rooms and areas in our living spaces that hold a special place in our hearts. Look around your house, and you'll find that subconsciously you've been favoring that place by placing pictures of your loved ones, statues, crystals, gemstones, etc. These objects carry a lot of significance on an emotional and on a spiritual level. So, on some level, a part of you has assigned a specific place for items of emotional and spiritual value. Such an area is often the best place to create an altar.

To start, you need to make known what you've been subconsciously doing. In other words, you need to acknowledge the importance of this shelf or corner. Then, while keeping your focus on this thought and with intention, cleanse your sacred space. Physically clean the area as you would normally clean it. After that, use rue or rosemary water to cleanse your space of negative energy.

Remember to keep your intentions focused on the sacred space you're creating and on who you are creating it for as you are cleansing it.

After having fully cleaned and cleansed your altar space, it is time to create the physical altar.

### 1. The Foundation

Cloth is the foundation of any altar. In addition to protecting the sacred space, it is a sign of the respect and honor you have toward the spiritual realm. If this is your first altar, a white cloth will work perfectly, although, later on, if you feel attracted to a particular design, symbol, or color, you can use that as a foundation.

### 2. Sacred Items

What you put on the altar is completely up to you. To a complete beginner, this can sound a bit vague and confusing as we're so often accustomed to clear instructions or dos and don'ts. The fact of the matter is that when it comes to your emotional and spiritual life, there **are** no clear instructions. It is all about what feels right to you. We can only provide you with guidelines, but you have to lead the way. If this feels scary to you, try to see the other side of the coin. There is no right or wrong. You can do anything you want as long as it aligns with you. Imagine the possibilities.

The sacred items you add can be anything from pictures and statues to m

ilagros to crystals. You can also add candles, flowers, and herbs. The rule of thumb is, as long as it makes you feel safe, comfortable, and in touch with your spirit and the spiritual beings you seek, it belongs on the altar.

# Tending to Your Altar

Caring for your altar is an integral part of keeping one. In doing so, you show your appreciation for the connection you have with your spiritual beings and your spiritual side. Because altars collect a lot of negative energy, especially if you do a lot of your healing near your altar, regular cleansing keeps the energy of your sacred space balanced.

This is why it is important to cleanse your altar at least once a month and whenever you feel the need to do so.

During this process, you may find that, in addition to the cleansing methods we mentioned above, the smoke that results from burning sage, palo santo, or copal is quite helpful in clearing out negative energy and restoring balance.

Don't forget to maintain focus on your intentions and, as you cleanse your space, remember to pay attention to the shift in the surrounding energy.

# End of Year Routine

The relationship between a person and their altar is a beautiful and sacred relationship. Many curanderos like to create an end-of-year routine as a way to strengthen and celebrate their relationships with their altars.

Spiritual end-of-year routines are very similar to other New Year's Eve traditions, like reflecting on our past year and making resolutions for the new one.

Some people choose to give thanks and show gratitude to their altar and spiritual beings for all the guidance and the support, others prefer to set intentions for their new year, and others prefer to look back at their past year and celebrate/honor their progress.

Your routine doesn't have to include or be limited to these three things. As you develop a relationship with your altar, your own unique end-of-year routine will come to you.

Keep an eye out for other routines that align deeply within you, such as routines that follow particularly tough periods or milestones or significant dates or events.

## The Day of the Messenger

One of the ways that we all acknowledge our cultures or beliefs is through designating some special dates to celebrate festivities. By marking these significant days on your calendar and engaging in celebration rituals alone or with a community, you'll be able to start deeply integrating curanderismo into your life.

For curandero, the most important celebration is "The day of the Messenger" or "El día del Guía." The day of the Messenger is December 21st which is known for many of us as the winter solstice.

The winter solstice marks the shortest day and longest night of the year. Curanderos believe that when the dark times are almost over, that is when we should be preparing for the good times to come and reconnect with our goals and aspirations.

As for the Messenger, it is the spirit of the Deer, a spirit that is believed to have existed since before Spain colonized the Americas. The spirit of the Deer was said to be able to tell you what will take place for someone in their coming year. That's why this day is a great time to reconnect with your life purpose and listen closely to any incoming messages from your spirit guides.

## How to Celebrate

Just like we all have Holiday traditions, and the same goes for New Year and Halloween, and you're more than welcome to celebrate the day of the Messenger in the way you see fit.

This could mean gathering with your closest friends, reflecting upon your past year, and setting your intentions for the future. It could also mean a special session in front of your altar, preparing a specific meal, or giving offerings of gratitude.

Most importantly, incorporating curanderismo in your day-to-day life, especially in these modern times where everything moves at such a fast pace, is about faith and dedication. While the rituals and amulets do possess power, this power comes from within you. Particularly, it is rooted in your faith and dedication. In other words, don't get so focused on the physical aspects of curanderismo that you forget about the spiritual side because these are its roots. Having said that, in the next chapter, you will find a selection of rituals and spells that will help you prepare many healing remedies, cure several illnesses, and soothe intense emotional pain.

# Chapter 10: Other Curanderismo Rituals

The way that Curanderismo approaches health is very different from modern medicine. The scientific approach relies on looking at the function of certain parts of the body and figuring out whether or not an organ, muscle, or system in the body is doing what it is meant to do. In most cases, a change in the way a part of the body operates is identified as the root cause of a problem. Then a doctor will try to resolve this matter in isolation to relieve the patient of the trouble they are experiencing. For instance, if a person is diagnosed with clogged arteries, a medical professional will perform surgery to expand the arteries and clear the blockage, or they may partially remove that artery and replace it with a new artery taken from a different place in the body. In milder situations, the doctor may suggest certain medications that will help thin the blood and also help clear the blockage. These medications are usually suggested with a certain diet plan, and through various tests, the blockage is evaluated and monitored.

Just like many other traditional treatments and alternative forms of medicine, in Curanderismo, functions of the body are not only limited to the organs. More importantly, different aspects of the human body are not only confined to doing what modern medicine defines them for. For instance, in many forms of traditional medicine, the heart not only pumps blood and creates a pulse in the body, but it is also responsible for the emotional quotient of a person, love, and spirituality. For this reason, the way the body is diagnosed and evaluated is very different from how it is done in Western medicine. Also, in Curanderismo and in many other traditional forms of healing, the ability to heal is seen as a special power that is given to certain individuals by God. While everyone may have the ability to heal - because all humans do have this ability - in some people, it is stronger than in others, and it appears they have been specially chosen to dedicate their lives to others by being healers.

However, the gift of healing alone is not enough, and even with this talent, individuals have to undergo an apprenticeship with a senior curandera to learn the different ways in which they can heal people and how they can harness resources to improve peoples' health. This internship involves a detailed study of plants and herbs and learning to understand how to interpret signs and symbols, so they come to understand the patient and even look into their future or past. However, even with all this training and knowledge, curandera's believe that God ultimately provides health and healing, and they act merely as vessels through which this divine energy is made available. They themselves do not claim any role in the process other than the fact that they were blessed with the ability to carry out this function. This is why most curanderas do not accept payment for their services, and any donations they accept are seen as donations to God and forms of charity rather than payments to the healer.

All of these factors combined have a large impact on the way that curanderas perform their treatments and the way they approach the entire concept of health and wellbeing. Let's look at a few more interesting ways in which Curanderismo can help you in your life.

# Curanderismo for Illness

As mentioned previously, the way that curanderas look at the human body and the way that traditional biology works are very different from what is seen in modern medicine and allopathic forms of medicine. One of the most prominent concepts in Curanderismo is the idea of food being inherently hot or cold and its effect on the body's temperature. This has nothing to do with the actual temperature of the food or drink, but it can be seen as the "personality" of that food. Moreover, certain processes in the body and certain things we do in life are also seen as *hot or cold activities*. For this reason, a person's diet is very important in Curanderismo. Often, a curandera will make dietary suggestions to help a person fight an illness, whether it is physical, mental, or spiritual. Certain food has its own energy, and this can also impact the overall balance in the body.

Food that is classified as having a "hot" nature will include such things as coffee, ginger, beef, fried foods, hard liquors, eggs, mustard, and lentils. Similarly, certain herbs and plants are also classified as either being hot or cold. Processes or activities considered hot would include things such as pregnancy, digestion, farming, and deep thinking. If a patient is suffering from illness and claims to also be battling in a difficult relationship, a stressful job, or has been facing many unforeseen circumstances, these can all be seen as triggers that may have influenced or created an imbalance in their bodily system.

On the other hand, cold things include activities such as childbirth, going through surgery, losing a loved one, and giving birth, among many other things. Also, certain things that we go through in our daily lives can also affect us negatively depending on the condition of our health and the severity of that activity. For instance, going out with wet hair or being exposed to a cold environment with wet hair is considered a cold activity. Walking on a cold floor with bare feet is considered a cold activity.

While this should not harm a person under normal circumstances, if the body is already weak, because the person is already suffering from an illness, these things can worsen the situation. Similarly, if the body is already in a hot state and someone eats or does something which also has a hot nature, it can cause an imbalance in the body and can lead to all kinds of complications. Also, sudden changes in the body that alter the state of the body from hot to cold or vice versa are quite dangerous. For example, if a body is already in a cold state and a person drinks iced water in that state, it will push the body into producing an excessive amount of heat to counter the cold water. This, in turn, will have a domino effect and bring about problems that are caused by too much heat.

The main reason for any illnesses identified by Curanderismo practitioners is an imbalance in the body and the energy within the body, which can be brought about by fatigue, stress, magic, or being surrounded by negative energy, among others. Through various f treatments, the curandera will try to restore balance and cast off any negative energy that might be surrounding the patient.

## Kinds of Illnesses

### Susto

This is one of the most common and most severe illnesses in which the soul leaves the body. The problem is characterized by behavior that modern psychology would classify as depression. The individual has problems sleeping, they are not very concerned about personal hygiene, they are withdrawn, they don't have an appetite, and they are generally disconnected from the world. Curanderas elaborate on this situation and say that what has happened is that the physical body has gone through an extremely negative and traumatic experience, so extreme that the soul within the body has been frightened and has left the body through fear of the situation. The soul is now separated from the body and will not return because it is scared. The solution is prayer, eating the right herbs, cleansing with holy water, visiting a curandero, and following their directions.

### Empacho

This is a digestive problem. The patient may be facing a blockage, excessive buildup of gas, or overall digestive problems. Many people also face cramps, a loss of appetite, and nausea. The most common causes for this are identified as eating food that has gone bad, eating too much food, eating something that you are not mentally comfortable with eating, or food getting caught somewhere in the digestive tract. Curanderas suggest that if a patient is suffering from these problems, they should start eating more mint and ginger to help the digestive process, combined with an increased intake of water. Also, the person should try not to spend too much lying around, and casual walks can help. Keeping the diet light and taking warm baths can also help to relieve this blockage.

### Caida De Mollera

This is a problem that affects infants and newborn babies and is known in western medical terms as a fallen fontanel. Babies don't have a fully developed skull, and the four major bones at the front of the skull are still forming. All these bones join at a central spot at the top of the head, and, in some cases, there can be a slight depression at this point because all four bones are curved slightly inwards. Other than the depression in the head, the child may have problems with digestion, colic problems, vomiting, and indigestion and may also have a fever. Western medicine is of the view that this is caused due to dehydration. However, Curanderismo practitioners believe it may be because the child was not suckled or taken care of, or the child had an accident or a traumatic experience. The healer can try to resolve this matter by holding some water in his or her mouth and then sucking on the depressed spot to create a suction and try to bring the bones back up again. Another form of treatment is where the baby is held upside down above a pot of warm water, and the curandera applies a solution onto the child's head, usually made from raw eggs and fresh soap. Another approach is to simply rub some raw egg on the dented area and let it dry up completely before it is washed off.

## Forms of Treatment

As discussed earlier, a curandera will rely on the most natural method of treatment, whether this means making changes to the diet or feeding the body with supplements such as various herbs and plants and naturally occurring substances. Just like in western medicine, these items are further processed in different ways to harness the specific characteristics of the resources being used.

One of the most common ways to treat patients is through the use of teas and herbal drinks. These are made by infusing the leaves, stems, or flowers of various plants in hot water. The curandera will advise the patient on how much and when these medicines should be consumed. Timing plays an important role in many kinds of treatments in Curanderismo.

In some cases, plants and herbs are cooked into solid natural oils to create balms and ointments used topically. Curanderas will also submerge various medicinal plants in strong alcohol to extract their medicinal properties and then cook the infused alcohol with sugar creating a thick syrup that patients can use. Pills are also found in traditional Curanderismo. However, this is a relatively recent development. When plants and herbs are ground into a fine powder, this powder is put into capsules making herbal medicine for patients to take just like regular western medication. Traditionally these pills would be made by hand into small beads or pellets, and then these would be taken. In some cases, the pellets are made from the thick sugary syrup that helps bind everything together and also adds a nicer flavor to the medicine. The types of herbs and plants that go into these processes naturally depend on the malady the patient is suffering from. However, all known diseases can be treated using this type of medication. People frequently use it for common problems such as headaches, indigestion, or seasonal allergies, as well as for more complicated and serious matters such as cancer, HIV, and diabetes. Some curanderas prefer to prepare the plants and herbs themselves for their patients, while others will resort to premade options that are easily available at traditional markets.

Plants, herbs, fruit, and vegetables all play an important role in the diet of the Mexican people. Many things that are used in Curanderismo are actually already a part of their daily diet. The thing they need to figure out is what they need and how much they need of it. For instance, things such as papayas, onions, garlic, cinnamon, and cumin are all frequently used in cooking. The same items can also be used for medicinal purposes. For example, papaya juice is good for cleansing and is often used to solve digestive problems, and even helps with headaches and mental discomfort. The main challenge with using these fruit and vegetables and other plants and herbs is when a patient is already using allopathic medicine and is looking to implement Curanderismo as well to help in the healing process. Some plants and herbs can have an adverse reaction to allopathic medicine if they are used in the incorrect quantities. Therefore, curanderas need to be careful when they are assisting someone who is already on another form of medication.

Certain items also have a religious and medicinal value in Curanderismo and in the Spanish culture in general. This will include things such as necklaces, amulets, wrist bands, pictures and statues of saints, the Christian cross, and certain perfumes and scents. Amulets are particularly common and are often prescribed to patients to be worn at all times. These can be made from a variety of items, including stones, metals, wood, and even plants and animal hides.

These items are believed to protect the wearer from negative external influences and help them protect their assets. Some people will decorate their home or their living room with a picture of a Saint or have a Christian cross hanging in a central part of the home, or they might have an aloe vera plant placed at the entrance of their home. All these objects are thought to not only have positive energy and a good influence on the premises, but they also help fight off negative energy and evil. Pregnant women are also advised to wear some form of metal when they are pregnant. This could be as small as a metal ring or maybe a metal necklace. The purpose is that it helps counter negative energy and helps protect the baby. It also helps protect the mother and the baby from the energy of the lunar eclipse, which is thought to cause birth defects and even miscarriages.

## Curanderismo for General Wellbeing

The Spanish culture is a mix of tradition, religion, healing, and social norms. As it covers such a large physical area, there are a lot of variations in what is considered Spanish culture, and things like food, music, and traditional healing vary a lot.

The most prominent aspect of healing that applies to all variations of the Spanish culture is healing through spiritual cleansing. As curandera see illness and problems in life as a result of imbalances in energy or due to evil spells and magic, the way to cure these ailments is to bring positivity into your life and counter any negative energy that you may have encountered or that may have been inflicted by someone else.

The other way to keep yourself healthy is through a healthy and balanced diet. Many things used in traditional medicine are also otherwise used in day-to-day food, such as onions, garlic, and cumin. Consuming a good diet will ensure that you are not only physically healthy – but also in good spiritual shape.

## Spiritual Baths

Spiritual baths are an important part of the healing process. In some cases, the bath itself can be the treatment, while in other cases, it is the first step toward preparing yourself for a cleansing. This is something that is carried out for all kinds of treatment, whether you are looking for relief from a physical, mental, or spiritual problem. As

Curanderismo is closely linked to religious rites and there is a strong spiritual side to this form of treatment, being clean both physically and spiritually is an important part of the recovery process.

Spiritual baths can be taken on your own, or they may be supervised by a curandera. For instance, the steam cleansing ritual in which a person goes into a small stone tent where the practitioner ladles holy water over volcanic rocks is a way to cleanse the person through steam and requires a teacher to perform it correctly. However, a person can also do this at home in their own bath by sitting in a tub of water with some Epson salts or some other herbs added to the water. The most important part of the spiritual bath is not how it is performed but the intention with which it is performed and how focused the person is on the spiritual side of the process. In most cases, there will be chanting going during a spiritual cleansing in a class setting or under the supervision of a senior. Some practitioners will choose to recite certain prayers, and as many people who follow this tradition tend to be Catholic Christians, they prefer to use The Lord's Prayer, among other prayers.

Those who are atheists and who do not believe in any particular deity can simply focus on themselves and think of the universe and talk out their thoughts and feelings and state their intentions to rid themselves of all negativity and evil and bring positivity into their lives through the act of cleansing.

A spiritual bath is also a form of treatment. For instance, when an egg cleansing follows the spiritual bath, the person will crack the egg and use this to produce a conclusion. Suppose the conclusion is that they are still suffering from negative influences and there is a spell or some form of negative energy they need to fight. In that case, the practitioner will advise them on what to do, and they will also continue to do spiritual cleansings. The cleansing itself is seen as a way to clear negativity from ones' life.

# Conclusion

In this book, the history of Curanderismo from its Aztec origins was discussed, and how ancient medicinal knowledge was combined Christian faith and other practices that shaped the way it is practiced to this day. In the first chapter, we discussed the different types of Curanderos and how it is important for the healer and the patient to have faith in this type of holistic healing system. We then introduced the main beliefs of Curanderismo practice that involve the healing of the mind, body, and spirit and how they are all connected by the universe's energy.

The third chapter focused on the most important plants and herbs used by a traditional Curanderismo healer and enlightened you to the various rituals and spells used to banish evil energy and dark forces. We explained how each plant works and where to find it. The fourth chapter was dedicated to ailments affecting the body. These included all the common physical illnesses from a sore throat to digestive and gut tract issues. We explained what causes these physical symptoms and how Curandero treats them.

The next chapter was aimed at spiritual cleansing and discovering its magical powers of healing. We mentioned the various tools and materials used by a Curandero to drive away evil energy. We also provided an example of rituals you can try on your own. The sixth chapter focused on the use of eggs in Curanderismo rituals and how they are important to absorb bad energy and serve as an indicator that a person has been afflicted with an evil force. We gave step-by-step instructions on how a Curandero performs a cleansing ritual using a raw egg and how they can find out if evil spirits exist.

In the seventh chapter, we focused on mal de ojo or the evil eye, a common belief found in many cultures around the world. Various countries create talismans or amulets to protect against the evil eye, which is believed to be cast on a person's possessions, health, or anything else which may attract an envious stare, which could be intentional or unintentional. We discussed who is most vulnerable to the evil eye and how to protect them against it. The eighth chapter was dedicated to a special type of spiritual ailment called susto or soul loss. We mentioned how a Curandero helps people with lost souls to restore them.

The ninth chapter discussed various tips and tricks of Curanderismo that you can use in your daily life. By keeping a few items close by, you'll be able to maintain your health physically, mentally, and spiritually. We also mentioned a few prayers recited in Curanderismo sessions to help keep you protected against negative energy and dark forces. In the final chapter, we mentioned additional rituals and spells used to heal various illnesses or emotional distress, from recovering from a broken heart to taking spiritual baths to heal your soul.

We hope you found this book useful in introducing you to the world of Curanderismo. Good luck on your healing journey!

# Here's another book by Mari Silva that you might like

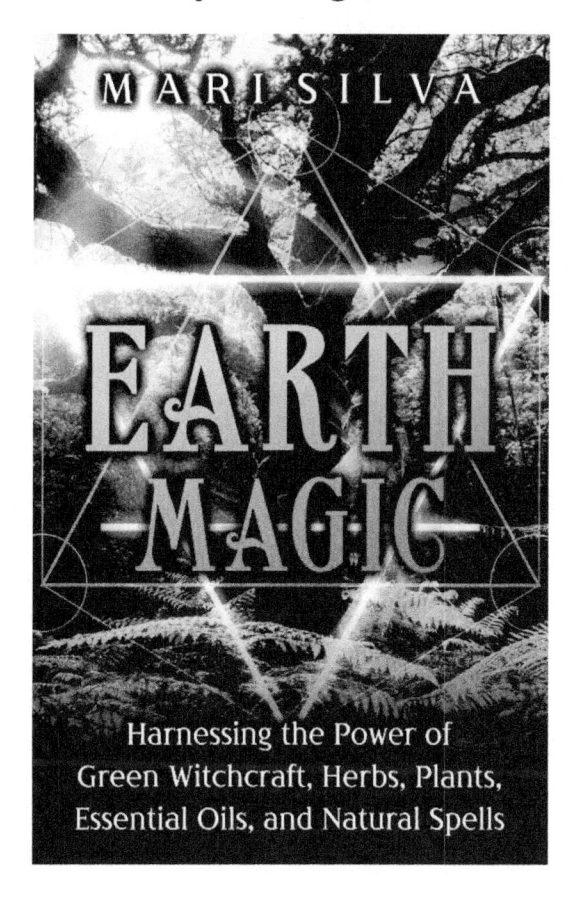

# Your Free Gift (only available for a limited time)

Thanks for getting this book! If you want to learn more about various spirituality topics, then join Mari Silva's community and get a free guided meditation MP3 for awakening your third eye. This guided meditation mp3 is designed to open and strengthen ones third eye so you can experience a higher state of consciousness. Simply visit the link below the image to get started.

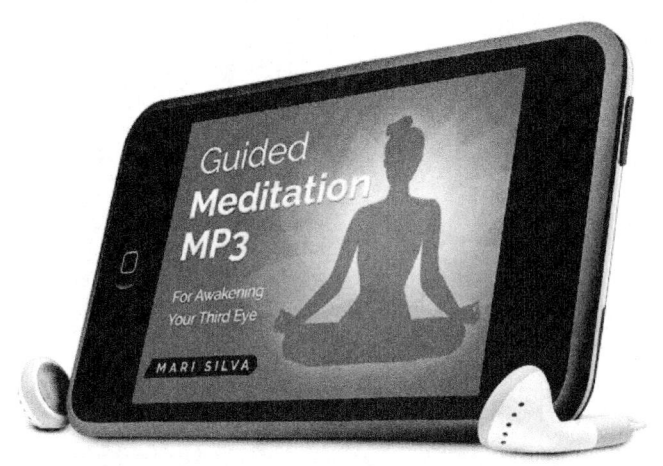

https://spiritualityspot.com/meditation

# References

Benner, M. (2018, July 17). Curanderismo, the Traditional Healing of Mexican Culture.

Fourdirectionswellness.Com.

https://fourdirectionswellness.com/2018/07/17/curanderismo-the-traditional-healing-of-mexican-culture

torres. (2019, June 21). Method and role as folk healer. Txstate.Edu.

https://www.txstate.edu/cssw/research-and-programming/cdvresources/windows/torres.html

Trotter, R. T., Chavira, J. A., & Robert T. Trotter II (Arizona Regents' Professor, Department of Anthropology, Northern Arizona University, Flagstaff, USA). (1997). Curanderismo: Mexican American folk healing (2nd ed.). University of Georgia Press.

Wigington, P. (n.d.). Curanderismo: The folk magic of Mexico. Learnreligions.Com. Retrieved from https://www.learnreligions.com/curanderismo-the-folk-magic-of-mexico-2562500

A curandera's garden of Mexican folk herbs. (2020, July 1). Moplants.Com.

https://moplants.com/a-curanderas-garden-of-mexican-folk-herbs

Carnation (Qu Mai). (2016, May 8). Whiterabbitinstituteofhealing.Com.

https://www.whiterabbitinstituteofhealing.com/herbs/carnation

Cavender, A. P., & Albán, M. (2009). The use of magical plants by curanderos in the Ecuador

highlands. Journal of Ethnobiology and Ethnomedicine, 5(1), 3.

Chilca dye plant. (n.d.). Ecotintes.Com. Retrieved from http://ecotintes.com/en/content/chilca-dye-plant

Cuya, M. H. (n.d.). Medicinal use of tobacco - takiwasi center. Takiwasi.Com. Retrieved from https://takiwasi.com/en/sinchi-negrito-tobacco.php

Northern tradition shamanism: The shamanic herbal: Plants of Frigga's handmaidens and

helpers. (n.d.). Northernshamanism.Org. Retrieved from

http://www.northernshamanism.org/plants-of-friggas-handmaidens-and-helpers.html

Rodríguez, C. (2021, June 15). Spiritual meaning of the colors of Carnations: Flower of love and passion. Ashepamicuba.Com; Ashé pa mi Cuba.

https://ashepamicuba.com/en/significado-de-los-colores-de-los-claveles

The teaching of Curanderismo traditional medicine through a free online course. (n.d.). Unm.Edu. Retrieved from http://news.unm.edu/news/the-teaching-of-curanderismo-traditional-medicine-through-a-free-online-course

(N.d.). Researchgate.Net. Retrieved from

https://www.researchgate.net/publication/281348129_Phytochemical_and_therapeutic_use_of_Baccharis_latifoliaRuiz_Pav_pers_Asteraceae

Blaesser, J. (2000). Curanderismo and Health Delivery Services. Portland State University

Library.

De Los Santos, L. (2020, April 14). Survival healing: Traditional Mexican remedies.

Southsideweekly.Com.

https://southsideweekly.com/survival-healing-traditional-mexican-remedies

Understand folk medicine's role in the prehospital care of many Mexican-Americans - JEMS.

(2009, December 1). Jems.Com. https://www.jems.com/training/understand-folk-medicines-role

(N.d.). Eric.Ed.Gov. Retrieved from https://files.eric.ed.gov/fulltext/ED270279.pdf

Limpias – energetic and spiritual Cleansing10-15-2014 - American botanical council. (n.d.). Retrieved from Herbalgram.org website: http://herbalgram.org/resources/herbclip/herbclip-news/2014/limpias-energetic-and-spiritual-cleansing

The Scarlet sage herb co.: Limpias for spiritual cleansing with napaquetzalli. (2019, February 10). Retrieved from Missionlocal.org website: https://missionlocal.org/event/the-scarlet-sage-herb-co-limpias-for-spiritual-cleansing-with-napaquetzalli

Discovering Greatness, L. L. C. (n.d.). Limpia Therapy. Retrieved from Discoveringgreatnessllc.org website: http://www.discoveringgreatnessllc.org/limpia.html

Ferraro, K. (2020, December 30). 10 easy ways to cleanse your home of negative energy.

Retrieved from Mindbodygreen.com website: https://www.mindbodygreen.com/0-4398/Easy-Way-to-Cleanse-Your-Home-of-Negative-Energy.html

Curandera, C., & View my complete profile. (n.d.). Curious Curandera. Retrieved from

Blogspot.com website: http://curiouscurandera.blogspot.com/2015/08/cleansings-in-curanderismo.html

Cleanse your aura with the power of eggs. (n.d.). Retrieved from Vice.com website:

https://www.vice.com/en/article/wnbxnn/cleanse-your-aura-with-the-power-of-eggs

Jackson, Y. (2012). Encyclopedia of multicultural psychology (Y. K. Jackson, Ed.). SAGE
Publications. https://play.google.com/store/books/details?id=AP1yAwAAQBAJ

Attanasio, C. (2015, March 11). Evil eye superstition: 5 ways 'Mal de Ojo' is cured in the Latin world. Latintimes.Com. https://www.latintimes.com/evil-eye-superstition-5-ways-mal-de-ojo-cured-latin-world-301842

Mal De Ojo - Top 10 Things about "Mal De Ojo" or the Spanish Evil Eye. (n.d.). Evil-Eye.Shop.

Retrieved from https://evil-eye.shop/mal-de-ojo.html

"Mal de ojo" or "Evil eye" - Nourish. (2021, March 2). 210Nourish.Com.

https://210nourish.com/mal-de-ojo-or-evil-eye

Mexico, N. (2021, May 26). El mal de ojo, The evil eye. Naatikmexico.Org; Na'atik Language & Culture Institute. https://naatikmexico.org/blog/el-mal-de-ojo-the-evil-eye

Radford, B. (2017, July 28). The evil eye: A closer look. Livescience.Com; Live Science.

https://www.livescience.com/40633-evil-eye.html

Woodman, S. (2018, March 13). What to know about the origins of Mexican folk healing.

Retrieved from Theculturetrip.com website:

https://theculturetrip.com/north-america/mexico/articles/everything-to-know-about-mexican-folk-healing

Curandera, C., & View my complete profile. (n.d.). Curious Curandera. Retrieved from

Blogspot.com website:

http://curiouscurandera.blogspot.com/2015/08/cleansings-in-curanderismo.html

Medical anthropology: Explanations of illness. (n.d.). Retrieved from Palomar.edu website: https://www2.palomar.edu/anthro/medical/med_1.htm

Curandera, C., & View my complete profile. (n.d.). Curious Curandera. Retrieved from

Blogspot.com website:

http://curiouscurandera.blogspot.com/2015/08/cleansings-in-curanderismo.html

Anderson, L. (2013, May 16). Curanderismo is alive and well in America. California Health Report. https://www.calhealthreport.org/2013/05/15/curanderismo-is-alive-and-well-in-america

Cocking, L. (2017, July 1). Meet Mexico's curandero healers keeping indigenous culture alive. Theculturetrip.Com; The Culture Trip. https://theculturetrip.com/north-america/mexico/articles/meet-mexicos-curandero-healers-enacting-surgical-miracles

Fernández, N. C. (2020, November 17). The Secrets of the Lodestone ≫ Attraction of triumph in the face of difficulties. Ashepamicuba.Com; Ashé pa mi Cuba. https://ashepamicuba.com/en/piedra-iman

García, B. (2020, September 18). Magic, Witchcraft, and Curanderismo: Let's talk about cultural appropriation. Aldianews.Com. https://aldianews.com/articles/culture/social/magic-witchcraft-and-curanderismo-lets-talk-about-cultural-appropriation

How to set and create your own altar. (2020, January 26). Hiplatina.Com. https://hiplatina.com/how-to-set-create-your-own-altar

Rue Water Recipe. (n.d.). Grouprecipes.Com. Retrieved from http://www.grouprecipes.com/101321/rue-water.html

Stiefer, A. (n.d.). El curandero actual: Preserving Indigenous Identity through Mexican Folk Healing's Chants. Shareok.Org. Retrieved from https://shareok.org/bitstream/handle/11244.46/90/6-THURJ-2016-Auston-Stiefer.pdf?sequence=3&isAllowed=y

Trotter, R. T., Chavira, J. A., & Robert T. Trotter II (Arizona Regents' Professor, Department of

Anthropology, Northern Arizona University, Flagstaff, USA). (1997). Curanderismo: Mexican

American folk healing (2nd ed.). University of Georgia Press.

Urban, D. (2020). Benefits of frankincense essential oil: 100% Pure therapeutic grade

frankincense and myrrh oil. Independently Published.

What is a Mexican Milagro? (n.d.). Zinniafolkarts.Com. Retrieved from https://zinniafolkarts.com/blogs/news/36153281-what-do-milagros-mean

Young, N. (2021, January 8). Limpias and herbal remedies to help kickstart the New Year. Hiplatina.Com. https://hiplatina.com/limpias-curanderas-new-year

TSHA. (n.d.). Retrieved from Tshaonline.org website: https://www.tshaonline.org/handbook/entries/curanderismo

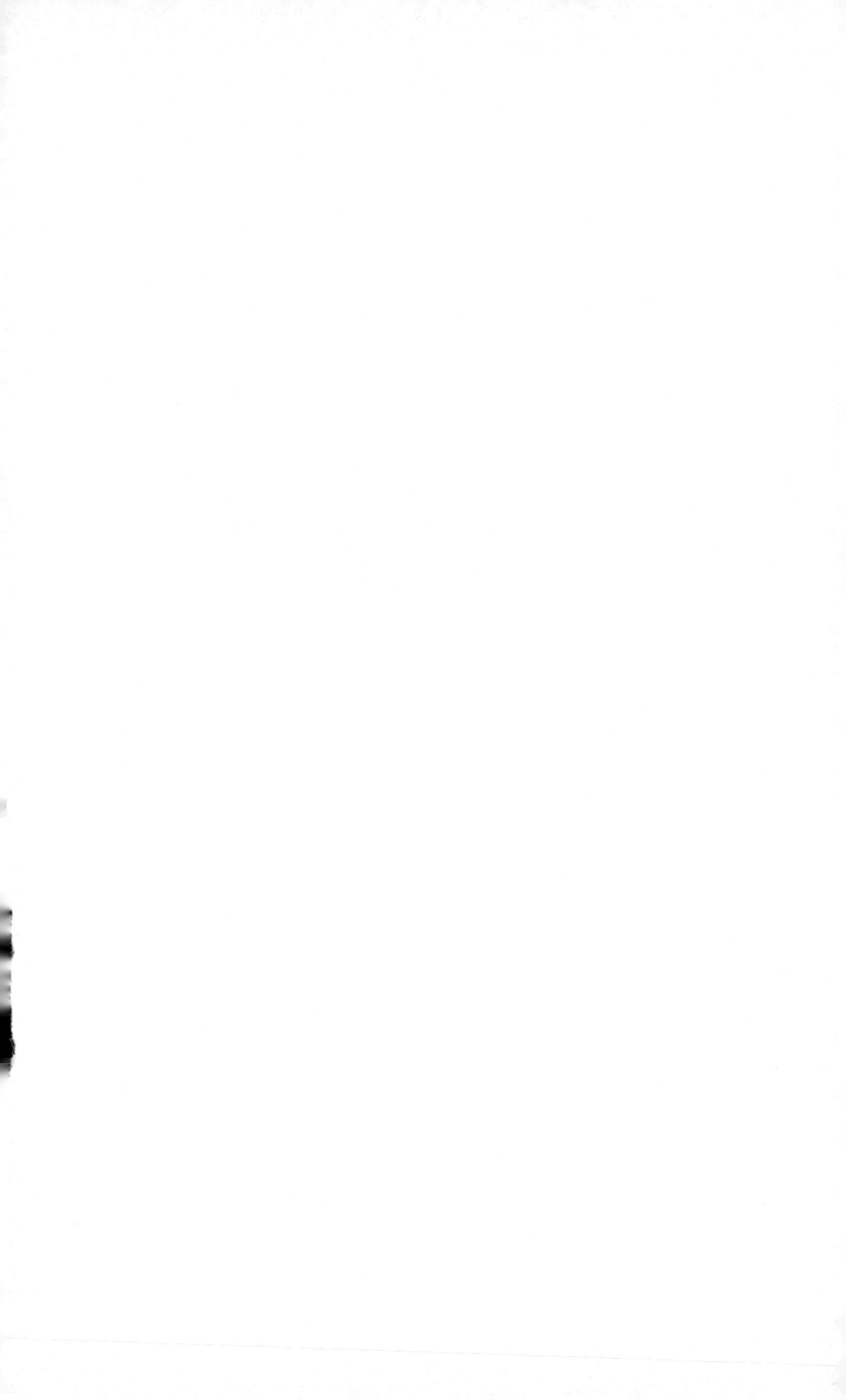